THE HARVARD UNIVERSITY PRESS FAMILY HEALTH GUIDES

Stroke and the Family

A NEW GUIDE

Joel Stein, M.D.

HARVARD UNIVERSITY PRESS
Cambridge, Massachusetts
London, England
2004

Library of Congress Cataloging-in-Publication Data

Stein, Joel.
  Stroke and the family : a new guide / Joel Stein.
    p. cm.—(The Harvard University Press family health guides)
  Includes bibliographical references and index.
  ISBN 0-674-01513-4 (cloth : alk. paper)—ISBN 0-674-01667-X (pbk. : alk. paper)
  1. Cerebrovascular disease—Patients—Family relationships. I. Title. II. Series.
  RC388.5.S785   2004
  362.196′81–dc22   2004052291

To my wife,
    Joanne, for her unconditional love and support

To my children,
    Daniel, Joshua, and Aliza, who bring joy to my life

Contents

STROKE AND THE FAMILY

Introduction

A stroke is actually a family illness.

McKenzie Buck, stroke survivor and psychologist

The diagnosis of stroke is a feared yet unfortunately common event. Despite its prevalence, however, both the lay public and medical professionals harbor many misconceptions about it. The very term "stroke" describes the way this disorder often occurs. Frequently an active, independent person is literally "struck down." Stroke is a sudden, life-altering event that often gives no warning of its approach.

This book is about life after a stroke, with an emphasis on providing information and resources for the family members of a stroke survivor. Knowledge can help loved ones obtain needed services, advocate for the survivor, and cope with the stresses that stroke creates for the entire family. Millions of stroke survivors and their families are living with a situation they never anticipated and feel ill-equipped to manage. It is easy to lose hope after a stroke, and society's attitudes about this disorder can make a difficult situation even worse. Unfortunately, many people in both the medical and the lay community believe that the useful, enjoyable phase of life ends when a stroke occurs. But there is good news: some stroke survivors are becoming more vocal about their experiences, sharing their stories and thus working to dispel these myths. Although stroke affects many different people in many different ways, plenty of individuals go on to live rich, satisfying lives after stroke, and they can serve as role models for the recently affected.

A person's response to stroke depends in substantial part on the individual's personality and character traits. Some people are used to controlling their own destiny, and so may react to a stroke by working vigorously to reestablish their independence and function. Others are more passive and may have a harder time mustering the resolve and determination to overcome the losses stroke imposes. I never cease to be amazed at the achievements of some of my stroke patients, who surpass my every expectation and achieve function I could not have reasonably expected them to attain. I have learned from these patients not to be too certain in my prognostications, and to always leave the door to hope ajar. Patients, families, and healthcare providers can all create self-fulfilling prophecies—for better or for worse.

There is a tendency among clinicians, patients, and families to focus on the limitations experienced after stroke. We all need to recognize that disability of one sort or another is pervasive in life. Many people live with pain from arthritis, vision or hearing loss, or a host of other physical limitations. People with disabilities cannot necessarily deny or change their limitations, but they can focus their attention on the many activities they can accomplish and enjoy. Indeed all of us, stroke survivors, families, and healthcare professionals, must focus our attention on stroke survivors' abilities rather than on their disabilities. The key to success after stroke is working to minimize limitations, accepting what we cannot change, and then moving on to the interesting and enjoyable parts of life.

What Is a Stroke?

Roberta, a seventy-four-year-old grandmother and retired schoolteacher, is having coffee with her daughter one afternoon when she suddenly announces, "I don't feel well." Her daughter notices that the right side of Roberta's face is drooping, and she is having a hard time swallowing her coffee. Over the course of a few minutes, Roberta begins to have trouble speaking and slumps over in her chair. Her daughter calls 911, and Roberta is rushed to a nearby emergency room. There the emergency room physician tells Roberta and her daughter that it appears Roberta is having a stroke. The two women are scared and confused. Is this really a stroke? Why wasn't there any pain or other warning signs? How could this happen so suddenly? Will Roberta be ok?

Unfortunately, Roberta's situation is very common. It is estimated that each year in the United States alone, 600,000–700,000 people suffer stroke. As a result, there are more than four million stroke survivors in this country today. Most adults, in fact, have family members or acquaintances who have had a stroke. Stroke is a leading cause of death in the United States and the number one cause of disability among adults. Despite its prevalence, however, many people have a very limited understanding of what a stroke is and what can be done about it.

A stroke is defined as permanent damage to an area of the brain caused by a blocked blood vessel or bleeding within the brain. There are a number of different ways stroke can occur, and the type of stroke will determine the appropriate treatment. All strokes share a common feature, however: they result in damage to one or more areas of the brain. Thus the aftereffects of stroke are primarily determined by the specific area(s) of the brain affected, rather than by the specific cause of the stroke.

Cerebral Infarction

The most common type of stroke is known as an "infarct," and it occurs when a portion of the brain loses its supply of blood. This can happen when a blood clot lodges within a blood vessel and blocks it, or when a blood vessel narrows to the point where blood can no longer flow through it. When an area of the brain is not getting enough blood, it fails to receive the oxygen and nutrients carried in the blood, and brain cells die from lack of these critical supplies. A stroke is similar in many ways to a heart attack, in which a portion of the heart loses its supply of blood, causing heart cells to die. One important difference is that the heart has an ample supply of nerves capable of providing pain sensation, whereas the brain has little ability to feel pain. As a result, many strokes are painless or have a relatively mild degree of pain. The absence of pain often leads people who are having stroke symptoms to delay obtaining medical care.

Cerebral Hemorrhage

Franklin is a sixty-three-year-old man with a history of prior polio and severe uncontrolled hypertension. Despite the advice of his physicians, he continues to maintain a highly active role in an extraordinarily stressful position. One day he exclaims to a staff member, "I have a terrific pain in the back of my head." He dies hours later of a massive cerebral hemorrhage. "Even His Family Unaware of Condition as Cerebral Stroke Brings Death to Nation's Leader at 63," reports the *New York Times* on April 13, 1945, after President Franklin D. Roosevelt's death.

The second major category of strokes are due to bleeding in the brain. These strokes are known as cerebral hemorrhages, and they account for about one-fifth of all strokes. In a cerebral hemorrhage, the bleeding in the brain puts pressure on the adjacent brain tissues and causes some of these cells to die. Because of the pressure created by the expanding area of blood within the brain, these types of stroke are commonly more painful than cerebral infarctions and may cause very sudden and severe headaches. Symptoms from cerebral hemorrhage are unpredictable, however, and some individuals have painless neurological symptoms indistinguishable from those of a cerebral infarction.

Warning Signs before a Stroke: Transient Ischemic Attacks (TIAs)

Jim is a sixty-four-year-old man with hypertension. He is overweight, sedentary, and smokes. At a business lunch with a client, he experiences some numbness and sudden clumsiness when moving his left hand. He continues his business lunch and feels relieved when his symptoms go away on their own after about five minutes. He almost forgets about the entire episode, but his wife insists that he contact their primary care physician. She read a magazine article that listed temporary clumsiness and numbness as possible warning signs of stroke. His physician finds that his exam is normal but tells Jim that he has had a "TIA." Jim is concerned—is he about to have a stroke? Can he do anything to prevent a stroke?

Transient ischemic attacks, or TIAs, are stroke-like episodes that resolve spontaneously, usually within minutes. TIAs result from temporary blockages to blood flow. Unlike in stroke, however, in a TIA the body is able to dissolve the blockage and restore blood flow before any permanent damage occurs. TIAs have traditionally been defined as stroke-like neurological symptoms that completely resolve within twenty-four hours. With the availability of better imaging techniques (especially magnetic resonance imaging, or MRI scans), it has become clear that sometimes events that appear to be TIAs are actually small strokes, with very rapid recovery. As a result, some physicians now consider TIAs to be stroke-like symptoms that completely resolve without any radiographic—that is, computerized tomography (CT) or MRI—evidence of stroke.

The most important aspect of TIAs is that they provide a warning to someone that a stroke may be imminent but is still preventable. The short duration and spontaneous resolution of TIA symptoms lead many individuals to ignore these events and not seek medical attention. In fact, people with TIAs are known to have a high risk of subsequent stroke and should obtain immediate medical evaluation. Treatment for TIAs varies with the cause, and may include aspirin or other medications, or occasionally surgery.

Acute Management of Stroke

In the past, the medical profession considered stroke an untreatable condition. When a person with stroke symptoms sought emergency care, he was assigned a low priority and often had to wait to be evaluated and treated. This has changed substantially in the past few years with the development of "clot-busting" or thrombolytic medications. These drugs, such as alteplase (TPA), can dissolve a blood clot that is causing a blockage. The brain is a fragile organ that cannot survive for long without a fresh blood supply bringing oxygen and other nutrients. For this reason, these treatments need to be given as quickly as possible. "Time is brain" is a common saying among neurologists treating acute stroke, because every minute counts. In order to increase the awareness of stroke as a treatable emergency, organizations such as the American Stroke Association (a division of the American Heart Association) and the National Stroke Association have established ongoing educational programs to alert people to the symptoms of stroke and the need to obtain prompt medical evaluation.

Stroke is often painless. Individuals suffering from the initial symptoms of stroke are sometimes inclined to "wait it out," hoping that the symptoms will resolve on their own. Obtaining immediate medical attention is the best way to prevent or limit the damage to the brain when stroke symptoms develop.

Stroke Symptoms

All stroke and TIA survivors and their families should be familiar with the symptoms of a stroke. It is important to recognize that stroke symptoms can vary substantially and may be mild. Someone who has had a stroke or TIA in the past may have very different symptoms with a new stroke. If in doubt, seek prompt medical evaluation. Some of the common symptoms of stroke include:

- Weakness on one or both sides of the body
- Loss of sensation
- Difficulty speaking
- Confusion
- Visual changes
- Drooling or difficulty swallowing
- Difficulty walking or loss of balance
- Dizziness or room spins

Emergency management of stroke continues to evolve rapidly. At present, the most widely available emergency treatment for stroke is TPA given through a vein ("intravenous," or "IV"). This treatment can be provided in most emergency rooms with appropriate expertise and experience. Generally speaking, these "clot-busting" treatments need to be started within the first three hours after a stroke. The earlier treatment is provided, the better, and research has shown that people receiving this treatment in the first 90 minutes after a stroke have greater benefits than those who receive treatment 90–180 minutes after a stroke. A number of important medical issues may prevent the use of thrombolytic medications, including a prior recent stroke, any history of abnormal bleeding, severe elevations in blood pressure, and recent surgery, among others. Because of these limitations, only a relatively small percentage of people who have a stroke actually receive this type of treatment.

Even when patients are carefully screened for administration of this drug, some can have bleeding in the brain as a complication from this powerful clot-dissolving medication. In other cases, the blockage of blood flow is not successfully dissolved, and the damage from the stroke is undiminished. Even when all goes well, significant neurological damage often still occurs even with treatment. Despite these limitations, thrombolysis is an important and effective treatment, and a major advance in the emergency management of stroke.

Some medical centers are currently studying the use of thrombolytic treatment given directly into the blocked arteries of the brain. In this treatment, a long, narrow tube known as a catheter is threaded through the blood vessels in the arm or leg into the neck, and the clot-dissolving medication is given right near the blood clot itself. Although this treatment is quite promising, it requires a large team of physicians who are available at very short notice. For this reason, its use is confined to a few large hospitals at this time.

Heparin is another medication commonly used for the treatment of acute stroke. Heparin prevents blood clots from growing larger and from forming new clots, but it does not actually dissolve existing clots. The goal with this treatment is to prevent progression of the stroke to a more severe stroke, or prevent a second stroke, but not to reverse the effects of the initial stroke. Heparin is typically given intravenously. It is commonly used when an individual with a stroke is not appropriate for TPA (for example, too much time has elapsed, or the patient has had recent surgery), and as a preventative measure after strokes resulting from blood-clot formation. Although intravenous heparin is widely used, there remains controversy about which specific subtypes of stroke are best treated with the drug. Research studies are ongoing.

Aspirin has been found to be useful in the treatment of acute stroke and is commonly used when the other treatments outlined above are not appropriate.

The medical management of acute stroke includes controlling any fever that develops, avoiding extremes of blood pressure (too high or too low), and treating any elevations of blood sugar resulting from diabetes. These actions appear to help limit the extent of the damage caused by a stroke.

In a small number of strokes, immediate surgery is beneficial. Severe brain swelling can accompany some strokes and can create life-threatening increases of pressure inside the skull. Removal of a portion of the skull, sometimes coupled with removal of some of the dying brain tissue, can allow room for the swelling of the brain. This drastic procedure is most commonly used for younger stroke patients with large strokes. The portion of skull removed may be temporarily implanted underneath the skin in the abdomen for later replacement. If the removed portion of skull is unavailable, a plastic "plate" is used to reconstruct the skull instead. A hockey-type helmet is often used to protect the head until the skull can be reconstructed.

In cases of large hemorrhages within the brain, the blood clot is sometimes surgically removed. This treatment, too, is generally reserved for life-threatening cases.

Family Response to Stroke

The first few days after a stroke are often very difficult for family and friends of the patient. Information provided by the hospital staff may be couched in medical jargon and be difficult to assimilate. Feelings of frustration and helplessness are common. How can families work with the medical team as partners to achieve the best outcome for the stroke survivor? Here are some practical suggestions:

Appoint a spokesperson. Designating one family member (or friend) to serve as the primary contact for the medical team will improve communication and clarify decision-making. The spokesperson can then regularly update other family members and relay any questions to the physician.

Establish daily contact with the physician. The family spokesperson should arrange for daily contact with the physician leading the team (commonly known as the "attending" physician), who can provide medical updates and answer questions as they arise.

Speak with the neurologist. In some cases, the neurologist will be the attending physician caring for the stroke survivor; in others, the neurologist will serve as a consultant to the attending physician. In the latter case, it is important to have direct contact with the neurologist, who is an expert in determining the cause of the stroke and can provide the most experienced opinion regarding prognosis. This contact need not be daily, but it should occur early after hospital admission, and then at least periodically during the hospital stay.

Contact the case manager. Most hospitals employ nurses or social workers as case managers to assist patients with discharge planning. The case manager plays a key role in determining the type and location of care the patient will receive after discharge. Since many stroke survivors require a stay in a rehabilitation facility before returning home, and many others require home services on discharge, the family should contact the case manager early in the hospital stay. This will allow the family to have early input into the discussion of the discharge plan and help make the best choices for the stroke survivor.

Educate yourself. Understanding the effects of stroke and the process of recovery and rehabilitation will make you a more effective advocate for your family member. See the Appendix for a list of resources.

Educate others. Other loved ones and friends may have less information than the most actively involved family members. Share your knowledge with them and encourage them to learn more about stroke. The American Stroke Association and National Stroke Association (see Appendix) provide short, easy-to-read pamphlets about stroke that may be helpful for family members.

Accept uncertainty. The first few days after a stroke are often filled with uncertainty. While the medical staff can provide their best estimates of prognosis, the reality is that sometimes a period of time must elapse before the outcome of a stroke is clear. Focusing on the immediate (for example, medical) and near-term (post-hospital rehabilitation) issues rather than on the long-term issues (for example, return to work, financial concerns) will allow time for the prognosis to become clearer and help prevent the stroke survivor's family from becoming overwhelmed.

Support the stroke survivor. Depending on the severity and type of stroke, the condition of the affected individual may range from fully awake and alert to, in severe cases, comatose with no ability to communicate at all. Even when it is uncertain if the stroke survivor is aware of your visits, providing comfort to an ill family member is important. Sitting with the stroke survivor, holding her hand, or stroking her hair may not be proven to help medically, but it provides emotional benefits for all involved.

Take care of yourself. Stroke is a crisis for all involved, and family members can easily fail to attend to their own needs during the hospitalization of the stroke survivor. Twenty-four-hour-a-day vigils in the hospital lead to exhaustion and exacerbate the emotional stress that family members commonly experience. Taking time for adequate rest, sleep, eating right, and exercise are important if family members are to preserve their own health and well-being.

2

Finding the Cause of a Stroke

Nicholas is a sixty-five-year-old recently retired accountant on a vacation cruise with his wife when he wakes up one morning with mild left-sided weakness. He is brought by helicopter to a hospital, where he is diagnosed with a cerebral infarction—a stroke. Within the first forty-eight hours he undergoes a CT scan, an MRI, an echocardiogram, and carotid ultrasound tests. While in the hospital he quickly regains most of his strength on the left side, but he wants to understand why all these tests were performed and what they show. What caused his stroke? Is he likely to have another one? What can he do to prevent future strokes?

Cerebral infarcts all result from interruption of blood flow to a portion of the brain, but they have a variety of specific causes. Determining the cause is particularly important when selecting treatment(s) to prevent another stroke. A number of tests are useful in determining the cause, though the actual selection of these tests will vary depending on the circumstances and availability. These tests include:

Computerized tomography (CT or CAT scan) of the brain. CT is a special computerized x-ray of the brain. CT scans can show the location and size of a stroke (see Figure 2.1). They can be performed quickly and are very good at finding any bleeding in the brain (see Figure 2.2). Damage from an infarct is not always visible when the scan is done soon after symptoms of a cerebral infarct develop, however.

Magnetic resonance imaging (MRI scan) of the brain. MRI provides very detailed pictures of the brain and does not involve any radiation. MRI scans typically take longer to perform than CT scans, but they may be better

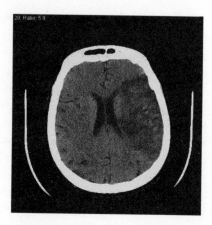

FIGURE 2.1   *Cerebral infarction.*
This CT of the brain shows a large infarct in the patient's left frontal and parietal lobes. The stroke appears darker than the surrounding brain. There is a small amount of bleeding within the stroke, visible as small areas that are lighter than the surrounding stroke.

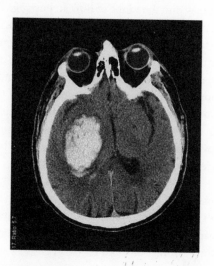

FIGURE 2.2   *Cerebral hemorrhage.*
This CT of the brain shows a large hemorrhage in the patient's right basal ganglia. The blood appears brighter than the surrounding brain tissue. A rim of edema (swelling) is seen around the blood and is darker than both the blood and the surrounding brain.

able to detect a stroke (especially an infarct) very early after symptoms develop. Certain people cannot undergo MRI, including those with pacemakers or other metallic objects in their body.

Magnetic resonance and computerized tomographic angiography. These techniques are used to provide pictures of the blood vessels supplying the brain. They are noninvasive and safe, and frequently provide sufficient information to direct treatment. In some circumstances conventional angiography is needed to provide even more detailed images.

Conventional angiography. In this procedure, detailed pictures of the blood vessels to the brain are taken by injecting a dye into the blood vessels via a special catheter (long, flexible tube). This is a more invasive procedure than MR or CT angiography and may carry some risk of adverse side effects, including stroke in rare cases.

Echocardiogram. In an echocardiogram, an ultrasound machine takes pictures of the heart using sound waves. These sound waves are at a high frequency and are beyond the range of human hearing. The sound waves bounce off the internal organs and are used to create a picture of the heart. There are two types of echocardiogram—a conventional or "transthoracic" echocardiogram, in which the recording head of the ultrasound machine is placed on the outside of the chest wall, and a "transesophageal" echocardiogram, in which the recording head of the ultrasound is swallowed and pictures are obtained from within the esophagus (the tube connecting the mouth with the stomach). Transesophageal echocardiograms provide more detailed pictures, and may be needed in certain circumstances to determine the cause of a stroke.

Electrocardiogram (ECG). Electrocardiogram, or ECG, is a routine recording of the heart's electrical activity. This is a simple and useful test for identifying damage to the heart, or an abnormal heart rhythm that may be responsible for a stroke.

Carotid ultrasound/transcranial doppler. This is another form of ultrasound that provides pictures and other information about the structure and functioning of the major blood vessels in the head and neck.

Holter monitor. Similar to an electrocardiogram, but obtained over a longer period of time (usually twenty-four hours), this test involves a special tape recorder that is carried by the patient. It can be useful in detecting abnormal heart rhythms that are intermittent and can cause stroke.

Blood tests for blood clotting. These tests check for abnormalities of blood clotting that can lead to stroke.

Lipid profile. This blood test, generally obtained after the patient has been fasting, provides information about fatty components of the blood, such as cholesterol and triglycerides, which can contribute to the risk of stroke. This test determines levels of high-density lipoprotein (HDL), the "good cholesterol" associated with a reduced risk of stroke, and low-density lipoprotein (LDL), the "bad cholesterol" that increases the risk of stroke and heart disease.

Types of Stroke

On the basis of the information obtained from these tests, physicians can usually identify the type and cause of the stroke. Ischemic strokes are often divided into several categories, depending on how the stroke occurs. Certain medical conditions may predispose individuals to particular types of stroke.

Embolic Stroke

Embolic stroke is caused by a clump of material traveling through the bloodstream and blocking a blood vessel in the brain. The substance causing an embolic stroke is most commonly a blood clot, though there are other substances that can "embolize" and cause stroke in rare cases, including pieces of cholesterol, fat from the middle of bones after a severe fracture, and even air. Blood clots can originate in a number of areas, as described below.

ATRIAL FIBRILLATION

A particularly common cause of blood clots forming in the heart is a condition known as "atrial fibrillation." In atrial fibrillation, the two smaller chambers of the heart, known as the atria, do not beat regularly and so cannot empty out all the blood they contain. Instead, the individual heart cells contract in an uncoordinated fashion, leading to inefficient pumping of the blood. This causes the blood to stagnate in the heart, allowing the formation of blood clots within the left atrium. These clots can break off and travel to the brain, causing a stroke. Warfarin (best known by its brand name, Coumadin) is the usual treatment for this condition, though aspirin is often used for individuals at low risk for stroke, and is a useful alternative for those unable to take Coumadin for medical reasons.

CARDIOEMBOLIC STROKE

Blood clots can originate in other parts of the heart, including the left ventricle, the main pumping chamber of the heart. This usually occurs when there is substantial heart disease and the heart is not pumping normally. In this case blood may have a chance to form a clot within the heart, resulting in a stroke if a piece of the clot breaks off and ends up in a blood vessel supplying the brain. The standard treatment is anticoagulation with Coumadin (warfarin) to prevent further clot development.

AORTIC ARCH EMBOLI

In recent years a relationship has been demonstrated between atherosclerosis (fatty deposits in the blood vessel wall) of a portion of the aorta, the main blood vessel carrying blood from the heart, and stroke. It is suspected that atherosclerosis in this area leads to an irregular surface inside the aorta, which allows clots to form and subsequently break off. These clots can then block a blood vessel in the brain and cause a stroke. Treatment typically involves Coumadin (warfarin) or aspirin to prevent another stroke.

PARADOXICAL EMBOLI

Before birth, there is normally an opening between the two smaller chambers of the heart (known as the atria). In most individuals this opening closes at birth, but it may remain open in some people throughout adulthood. This condition is usually asymptomatic. The opening is known as the "foramen ovale," and when it remains open after infancy, it is known as a "patent foramen ovale," sometimes abbreviated as PFO. In individuals with normal heart anatomy, the blood coming back from the body travels through the lungs before being pumped back to the head and body. The small blood vessels in the lungs function as a sort of filter, "catching" any blood clots that may be present. This filtering function prevents any of these clots from traveling to the brain and causing a stroke. In individuals with a PFO, however, some of the blood returning from the body bypasses the lungs and is pumped directly back to the brain and body. If there is a blood clot contained in this blood, it may be carried to the brain and cause a stroke. Fortunately, blood clots traveling in the blood are a relatively uncommon event, so individuals with a PFO may never have any symptoms. Nonetheless, PFO is increasingly recognized as a cause of stroke, particularly in young people without other known causes for stroke. Treatment for a PFO may include anticoagulation (Coumadin) or closure of the opening. This closure can now be performed in some centers via a catheter, thus preventing open-heart surgery.

Atherothrombotic Stroke

Atherothrombotic strokes are those that occur as a result of a blockage of the blood vessels supplying blood to the brain. These are often divided into two distinct subgroups: blockages of the small blood vessels within the brain ("lacunar strokes") and blockages of the large vessels supplying the brain.

LACUNAR INFARCTS

Blockages of the small blood vessels within the brain can cause small strokes known as lacunar infarcts. Because of their small size, the effects of these strokes vary widely. Some lacunar strokes do not cause any symptoms and are only detected incidentally on a CT or MRI of the brain. Others occur in critically important areas of the brain and can lead to severe weakness of an entire side of the body. This type of stroke is strongly associated with hypertension. Blood pressure control and anti-platelet medications (such as aspirin) are the main preventative measures.

CAROTID ARTERY NARROWING AND BLOCKAGE

Blockage ("stenosis") of the large blood vessels in the neck, the carotid arteries, can cause stroke (see Figure 2.3). These blockages often develop gradually over a long period of time and can be detected through ultrasound testing. Surgical treatment for these blockages is known as an "endarterectomy" and consists of removal of the inner layers of the blood vessel creating the blockage. This surgery is effective in preventing future strokes but does carry some risk of stroke at the time of surgery. Having the surgery performed by an experienced surgeon at a center that does a large number of these procedures appears to be the best approach for minimizing this risk. Complete blockage of one of these blood vessels (known as a carotid "occlusion") is generally not amenable to surgery, and in such cases medications are used to reduce the risk of future stroke.

Recently, experimental devices have been developed to keep these arteries open without surgery. These devices, known as "stents," are placed inside the blood vessel through a nonsurgical procedure in which a long, thin, flexible tube (catheter) is threaded through the blood vessels starting in the arm or groin area. The stent, a tubular, expandable wire mesh device, is then placed in the area of blockage using the catheter, and expanded to hold the blood vessel open. This treatment remains experimental and is being studied at a number of centers. It is not suitable for all blockages, depending on the specific anatomical issues in each case. Medical treatment with Coumadin (warfarin) or antiplatelet medications such as aspirin or clopidogrel (Plavix) is sometimes used for lesser degrees of blockage, while the patient awaits surgery, or in individuals who are unable to undergo surgery. Surgery remains the most common treatment at present for moderate to severe blockages.

VERTEBROBASILAR STENOSIS

In addition to the two large carotid arteries on each side of the neck, there is a third major artery supplying blood to the brain—the basilar artery. The basilar artery receives its blood from two arteries in the neck known as the vertebral arteries. Like the carotid arteries, any or all of these arteries may become blocked over time. Unfortunately, because of their location, these arteries are not presently amenable to surgical treat-

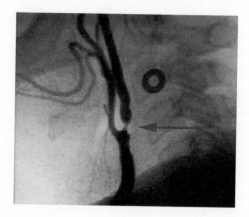

FIGURE 2.3   *Carotid stenosis.*
The carotid arteries are shown in black in this angiogram. The narrowing
(stenosis) of the internal carotid artery is visible at the arrow.

ment. Medical treatment (with aspirin, for example) is the usual approach. As with carotid artery blockages, research on the use of stents to
hold the artery open is ongoing.

INTRACRANIAL STENOSIS

Blood vessels within the head can become progressively narrowed and
blocked, leading to the development of a stroke. Because of the location
of these blood vessels within the skull, they cannot be corrected by surgery. The usual treatment in this situation is an anticoagulant, such as
Coumadin (warfarin), or an antiplatelet medication, such as aspirin or
Plavix (clopidogrel).

CRYPTOGENIC STROKE

"Cryptogenic" is an elegant way of saying "unknown cause," and cryptogenic strokes are those for which no cause can be determined. Despite
the extensive diagnostic tests undertaken, a cause remains unidentified
for a significant number of strokes. Treatment of these strokes generally
involves antiplatelet medications, such as aspirin or Plavix (clopidogrel),
or Coumadin (warfarin).

Other Types of Stroke

WATERSHED INFARCTS AND ANOXIC ENCEPHALOPATHY

Any condition that leads to severely reduced blood pressure and blood flow can result in a stroke or brain damage. Examples of this include a fall in blood pressure that occurs during surgery, or temporary loss of blood flow during a cardiac arrest. When blood flow is substantially reduced, the strokes that result commonly occur in the boundaries between areas of the brain supplied by different arteries, rather than being centered in the area supplied by a specific artery. These strokes are often referred to as "watershed" infarcts, because they occur at the boundary between two areas of blood circulation, or "watersheds." In some cases, such as cardiac arrest, blood flow to the entire brain is compromised simultaneously. In these cases, damage is more diffuse throughout the brain, with some areas more sensitive to the injury than others. Failure of blood or oxygen flow to the entire brain is known as an "anoxic" injury (meaning lack of oxygen). Memory problems are often very prominent in these type of injuries and may be the major long-term effect.

ARTERIAL DISSECTION

Blockage of a blood vessel leading to a stroke can be caused by a separation that forms between the inner layer of a blood vessel and the outer layers, resulting in a blockage in the artery. This is known as an arterial dissection. This is a cause of stroke in otherwise young, healthy individuals who do not have the usual risk factors for stroke. Arterial dissection often occurs after a minor injury, often one involving twisting or bending of the neck, though sometimes no injury can be identified. Chiropractic manipulation of the neck has been found to result in arterial dissection in a small number of people. Some individuals appear to have a genetic predisposition to this type of stroke, but the exact reason a dissection occurs often remains unknown. Treatment involves anticoagulation with heparin and then Coumadin (warfarin) for a period of time.

HYPERCOAGULABLE STATES

Several abnormalities of blood clotting cause the blood to clot (coagulate) more easily and quickly than normal. These disorders are known as "hypercoagulable" conditions. Most are genetic and are frequently asymptomatic. In a minority of individuals, however, this increased tendency to form clots can lead to a stroke. Some hypercoagulable states develop as the result of an acquired condition rather than a genetic one. These include antiphospholipid antibody syndrome, in which the body forms antibodies against itself, and the hypercoagulable state frequently present in people with cancer. Treatment for hypercoagulable conditions varies according to the severity and type of disorder and often involves anticoagulants such as Coumadin (warfarin).

The use of oral contraceptives can increase the risk of clotting somewhat and is implicated as a cause of stroke in some young women. For this reason, the use of oral contraceptives may be inadvisable in young women who have suffered a stroke, even if they were not using these medications at the time of their stroke. The combination of smoking and older age (for example, being in your forties versus your twenties) appears to increase the risk of stroke associated with oral contraceptives.

MIGRAINOUS STROKES

Migraine headaches are very common, affecting millions of Americans. In a very small number of cases, migraine headaches can be associated with stroke in a young adult. This is believed to be caused by severe spasm of the blood vessels, leading to a blockage of blood supply to a portion of the brain. The use of oral contraceptives in young women with migraine headaches seems to increase the risk of this type of stroke.

STROKES CAUSED BY ILLICIT DRUG USE

Certain illicit drugs, most notably cocaine and amphetamines, are known to cause ischemic strokes or hemorrhagic strokes in a small number of people.

CEREBRAL VENOUS THROMBOSIS

This relatively rare type of stroke involves not the blood vessels bringing the blood to the brain (arteries) but rather the blood vessels that drain the "used" blood away from the brain (veins). In cerebral venous thrombosis, a clot develops within these veins, causing the blood to "back up" within the brain. This results in a stroke, which can develop superimposed bleeding in some cases (see "Hemorrhagic Conversion"). The treatment for this type of stroke is anticoagulants such as heparin and Coumadin.

Cerebral Hemorrhage

Cerebral hemorrhage, or bleeding in the brain, has several causes. Although the effects of cerebral hemorrhage resemble ischemic stroke in many ways, their causes are quite distinct.

HYPERTENSIVE HEMORRHAGE

Elevated blood pressure can cause rupture of a blood vessel within the brain, known as a hypertensive hemorrhage. The worse the hypertension, the higher the likelihood of such a hemorrhage occurring. In a famous example, Franklin D. Roosevelt died in office of a cerebral hemorrhage caused by uncontrolled hypertension. Fortunately, many medications to control high blood pressure are now available, allowing effective blood pressure control in the vast majority of individuals with hypertension.

CEREBRAL AMYLOID ANGIOPATHY

In some older individuals, an abnormal protein is deposited in the walls of the blood vessels in the brain, causing the blood vessels to become fragile. This can result in rupture of the blood vessels and cerebral hemorrhage. This condition, known as cerebral amyloid angiopathy (CAA), can be difficult to diagnose with certainty in some cases. Unfortunately, there is no effective treatment for this disorder at the present time, and recurrent hemorrhages are possible. Avoiding medications known to increase the risk of bleeding, such as aspirin or Coumadin (warfarin), as well as alcohol is advised. Good control of hypertension, if present, is also advisable, since elevated blood pressure may increase the risk of a hemorrhage due to cerebral amyloid angiopathy. Research on possible treatments for this condition is ongoing (see Appendix).

ANEURYSMS

There are several types of malformations of the blood vessels that can cause a hemorrhagic stroke. One of the more common types is an aneurysm, which is an out-pouching of one of the larger arteries in the brain (see Figure 2.4). Aneurysms tend to run in families and can be asymptomatic for many years. Larger aneurysms have a greater risk of bursting and typically cause bleeding around the brain rather than inside it. This

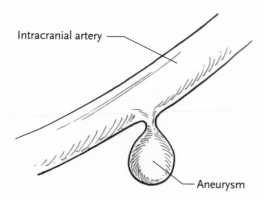

Intracranial artery

Aneurysm

FIGURE 2.4 *Cerebral aneurysm.*
This diagram shows an outpouching of the blood vessel (aneurysm), which can rupture and lead to bleeding around the brain.

type of bleeding is known as a subarachnoid hemorrhage. The effects of a ruptured aneurysm vary widely, ranging from severe headache without any other neurological problems to coma and even death. Surgery to "clip" the aneurysm or catheter placement of small detachable wire coils to clot off the aneurysm are the usual treatments. In some cases, the bleeding around the brain irritates the blood vessels of the brain, which can spasm so severely that blood supply to an area of the brain is interrupted, and a stroke occurs. Medications such as nimodipine (Nimotop) are used to prevent this complication of subarachnoid hemorrhage, though they are not always effective.

ARTERIOVENOUS MALFORMATIONS (AVMS)

Another type of blood vessel malformation is an arteriovenous malformation, or AVM (see Figure 2.5). An AVM is a complicated tangle of abnormal arteries and veins in the brain that may grow over time. Sometimes the growth of the AVM can cause symptoms by itself, without actually bleeding. Commonly, however, these malformations bleed into the brain owing to the fragility of the abnormal blood vessels contained in the AVM. If the hemorrhage is large and the AVM was not previously identified, it may be difficult to find the AVM on the initial scans of the brain, since the blood may obscure it. If AVM is suspected, follow-up

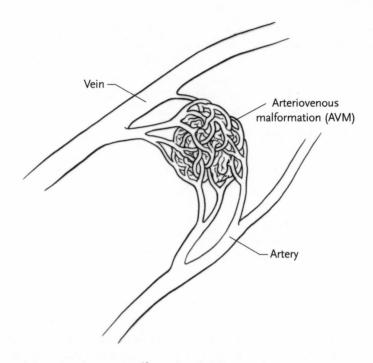

FIGURE 2.5   *Arteriovenous malformation (AVM).*
This diagram shows a tangle of abnormal fragile blood vessels connecting an
artery with a vein in the brain.

scans are often advised in order to examine the brain after the hemorrhage has been reabsorbed. Treatment for AVMs also involves the use of
catheter-delivered coils to reduce the size of the AVM or block off the major blood vessel "feeding" (providing blood to) the AVM. Surgery may
also be used to remove all or part of the AVM. Finally, radiation therapy
can be used to shrink the AVM. A combination of these techniques is
sometimes used, with coils or radiation used to reduce the size, followed
by surgery to remove the remaining AVM.

HEMORRHAGIC CONVERSION

In some cases, a stroke can start out as an infarct, but then bleeding
occurs into the area of the stroke. This is known as a "hemorrhagic conversion" of the stroke. The superimposed hemorrhage may be large or

small. Small hemorrhages are often of little significance, since they are in the middle of an area of brain tissue that has already been irreparably damaged. In larger hemorrhagic conversions, however, the hemorrhage may cause as much or more damage than the original stroke. Hemorrhagic conversion usually occurs in larger strokes and may be related in some cases to the use of anticoagulants (heparin or Coumadin). Often no specific treatment is needed, though anticoagulants are commonly discontinued when hemorrhagic conversion occurs. The risk of hemorrhagic conversion exists primarily within the first few weeks after stroke and is uncommon afterward.

Stroke-Like Conditions

A number of conditions affect the brain and can cause symptoms similar to those seen after stroke. These include any condition that results in a localized injury to the brain. Brain tumors, both benign (such as a meningioma—a tumor of the lining of the brain) and malignant (arising in the brain, or coming from another part of the body) frequently cause stroke-like problems. These most commonly have a more gradual onset—weakness that gets worse over a period of weeks, for example—rather than the sudden onset more typical of stroke. Multiple sclerosis can produce symptoms that are similar to those resulting from stroke. Trauma to the brain (for example, from a car accident) often produces more diffuse damage to the brain than stroke does, and tends to result in a different though overlapping set of problems. A detailed discussion of traumatic brain injury is beyond the scope of this book (see Appendix for resources).

SUBDURAL HEMATOMA

A subdural hematoma is a collection of blood between the brain and the skull (see Figure 2.6). Hematomas can result from falls or other injuries, an abnormal tendency to bleed (as when someone receives Coumadin in excessive doses), or occasionally without a clear cause in the elderly. The pressure exerted by this collection of blood affects the brain's functioning, causing confusion and sometimes weakness. Surgery may be necessary in some cases to remove the blood and relieve the pressure on the brain.

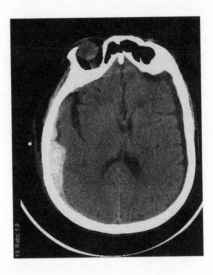

FIGURE 2.6   *Subdural hematoma.*
The collection of blood between the brain and the skull (subdural
hematoma) in this CT scan appears as a lighter-colored crescent-shaped area
on the left.

BRAIN ABSCESS

Like any other organ of the body, the brain can develop infections. A collection of pus can develop in severe brain infections, known as a brain
abscess. Brain abscesses can result from dental infections, heart valve
and bloodstream infections, or other infections elsewhere in the body.
Headache and fever are common, and symptoms often develop more
gradually than in a stroke. Treatment includes surgical drainage of the
infection and intravenous antibiotics. Once the brain abscess is treated,
the aftereffects are often very similar to those of stroke.

Most stroke-like conditions can be distinguished fairly easily from
stroke by the medical history and by CT or MRI images. From the perspective of patients and their families, stroke-like conditions present
many of the same challenges as stroke and may pose some additional
challenges as well. In the case of brain tumors, there may be a need for

surgery, followed by radiation and/or chemotherapy in some instances. In cases where these conditions are not curable (unfortunately, still a common situation), the likelihood of progression of the cancer creates a very different and complex set of issues beyond those caused by the neurological damage itself.

3

Stroke Prevention

Roberta, whom we met in the first chapter, is found to have a stroke caused by a blockage affecting her left middle cerebral artery. Further evaluation reveals that she has an irregular heartbeat, known as atrial fibrillation. After discussing the risks and benefits of treatment with Roberta and her family, her doctor starts her on Coumadin (warfarin) to reduce the risk of any future strokes. Is this the best treatment for stroke prevention? What else can Roberta do to reduce her risk of another stroke?

Prevention of Ischemic Stroke

Medications

Stroke prevention through the use of medication is a rapidly evolving area, and new data are becoming available all the time. This discussion is intended to provide general information rather than a guide to specific care. Several broad classes of treatment are currently available and will be discussed as categories.

ANTIPLATELET MEDICATIONS

Platelets are small particles that circulate in the bloodstream and help form blood clots to prevent or stop bleeding. Since blood clots are an important factor in causing strokes, medications that interfere with platelet function can be useful in preventing stroke. A number of medications have been developed for this purpose, including aspirin, an aspirin/dipyridamole combination (Aggrenox), clopidogrel (Plavix), and ticlopidine (Ticlid). All these medications have been found to be effective in reducing the risk of a second stroke and are also useful in individuals at high risk of a first stroke (for example, people who have had TIAs). While generally well tolerated, aspirin (and Aggrenox, which contains aspirin) can cause stomach upset or even ulcers in some people. Ticlopidine, and less frequently Plavix, can cause blood abnormalities in some people. As with any medication intended to interfere with blood clotting, antiplatelet medications do increase the risk of abnormal bleeding somewhat. But they are less risky in this regard than certain other medications, such as Coumadin (warfarin). Antiplatelet medications are generally the drugs of choice for prevention of lacunar strokes (those resulting from blockage of the small blood vessels) and strokes without a clear cause. Overall, these are effective, important, and well-tolerated medications for the prevention of stroke.

WARFARIN (COUMADIN)

Warfarin, commonly referred to by its brand name, Coumadin, is a powerful anticoagulant (sometimes known as a "blood thinner," a misleading term) that interferes with blood-clot formation. Coumadin requires careful adjustment, as too small a dose is ineffective, whereas too large a dose can be quite dangerous. Individual dose requirements vary widely and dosing must be individualized. Blood must be tested frequently—often weekly until a stable dose is achieved. This blood test, known as a "Protime," measures the time required for a component of blood clots to form and is usually reported as an International Normalized Ratio, or INR. INR target values vary with the cause of the stroke and may be individualized to some extent. Physicians prescribing Coumadin determine this range on the basis of the diagnosis, and take into consideration the increased risk of bleeding at higher INR values, as well as the risk of insufficient protection against stroke at lower INR values.

The Coumadin dosage required to keep the INR at the right level may vary over time. Changes in diet and other medications can require significant changes in Coumadin dose. For this reason, periodic monitoring through blood tests is required as long as someone is taking Coumadin. Changes in dosage are commonly required.

Coumadin is the preferred preventative treatment for strokes that are caused by blood clots forming in the heart, such as atrial fibrillation. It is often used for other types of stroke as well, though controversy persists regarding which patients should receive Coumadin versus antiplatelet medications. Coumadin is sometimes combined with antiplatelet medications in selected circumstances.

Family members should be alert for any symptoms of abnormal bleeding in a person on Coumadin, such as severe or repeated nosebleeds, bleeding from the gums, abnormal bruising, vomiting blood or brown material (blood turns brown in the stomach), or bloody or tarry black stools (blood turns black and tarry in the intestines). A sudden or severe headache or unusual pains in the abdomen or lower back can sometimes be due to internal bleeding and should be evaluated by a physician. Abnormal bleeding can occur even if a person's dose of Coumadin is appropriate, though it is most common when the dose is excessive.

People taking Coumadin are advised to use an electric shaver rather than a razor. Aspirin should be avoided unless specifically prescribed by a physician. Over-the-counter medications may interact with Coumadin and should be discussed with a physician before use. Alcohol usage should be minimized. Many medications can affect the body's metabolism of Coumadin, necessitating a change in dose. Any change in medications should be discussed with the physician monitoring and adjusting the Coumadin dose.

Certain foods contain large amounts of vitamin K, a substance that counteracts the effects of Coumadin. Small amounts of foods containing vitamin K are not a problem and are in fact a necessary part of a well-balanced diet. But eating large amounts of vitamin K–containing foods can render Coumadin treatment ineffective. Foods high in vitamin K should be eaten in moderation and in consistent amounts. Abruptly increasing or decreasing the level of vitamin K in the diet can render the dose of Coumadin too high or too low. Some herbal supplements include vitamin K–containing ingredients and may pose a hazard. A comprehensive listing of vitamin K content of a broad range of foods is available on the Dupont (makers of Coumadin) web site (see Appendix). The following is a list of some commonly eaten foods that are high in vitamin K:

Beet greens
Brussel sprouts
Collard greens
Dandelion greens
Endive

Kale
Parsley
Scallions
Spinach
Turnip greens
Watercress

The following foods contain moderate amounts of vitamin K:

Asparagus
Avocado
Broccoli
Cabbage
Mustard greens
Spinach

HEPARINS

Heparins are anticoagulant (blood-clot preventing) medications that come in several varieties. Conventional heparin (generally known just as "heparin" or "unfractionated heparin") is available only by injection, and may be given as a continuous intravenous medication or via two or more injections under the skin each day. Heparin is often used as a short-term treatment immediately after a stroke, or in lower doses to prevent blood-clot formation in the legs after stroke. Its use has been substantially supplanted by a new class of medications known as "low molecular weight heparins." These include dalteparin (Fragmin), enoxaparin (Lovenox), tinzaparin (Innohep), and others. These newer (and more expensive) medications are given as injections once or twice daily, and are at least as effective as heparin, safer, and easier to administer and monitor. They are generally used for short-term treatment for stroke prevention; individuals needing long-term anticoagulant medication are usually switched over to Coumadin instead. Heparins are sometimes employed for short-term management of individuals with severe blockages of a carotid artery who are scheduled for surgery in the near future.

CHOLESTEROL-LOWERING MEDICATIONS ("STATINS")

The "statin" drugs include a number of closely related medications such as simvastatin (Zocor), pravastatin (Pravachol), lovastatin (Mevacor), atorvastatin (Lipitor), rosuvastatin (Crestor), and others that are used to lower cholesterol levels in the blood. These medications have been found to be helpful in reducing the risk of stroke and are increasingly used for this purpose. Interestingly, these drugs appear to lower the risk of stroke even in people with "normal" cholesterol levels—a phenomenon that has not yet been fully explained. These medications are commonly used in combination with one of the other medications (such as aspirin) described above to reduce the risk of stroke.

ANTIHYPERTENSIVE MEDICATIONS

Many medications are used to lower blood pressure, and these are often used in combination. Some common medications and their features are listed in Table 3.1.

Stroke Risk Factors

Stroke risk factors are individual behaviors or characteristics that allow physicians to determine an individual's risk of having a stroke when compared with the general population. Some risk factors are stronger than others—for example, smoking is a stronger risk for stroke than ethnic background. Some risk factors can be changed (by quitting smoking, for example), whereas others (like age) are beyond our control. While risk factors are very helpful in choosing treatments for stroke prevention, they do not actually tell us who will and who will not have a stroke. Everyone has at least a small risk of stroke, and no one, regardless of how many risk factors, is guaranteed to have one. The value of risk factors is that they allow us to identify individuals at higher risk of stroke and develop a strategy to reduce that risk.

Modifiable Risk Factors

In many ways, modifiable risk factors are the most important ones, because we can change or sometimes eliminate them. Even individuals with nonmodifiable risk factors (for example, a strong family history of stroke) can reduce their overall risk by focusing on the modifiable risk factors (for example, starting to exercise). Not all modifiable risk factors can be easily changed. For example, a person may recognize that obesity

Table 3.1   Antihypertensive Medications

Class of Medication	Medications	Key Features	Common Side Effects
Diuretics	Hydrochlorthiazide (Hydrodiuril)	"Water pills"—cause the body to produce more urine	Frequent urination, low potassium levels
Beta blockers	Atenolol (Tenormin) Metoprolol (Lopressor) Propranolol (Inderal) Nadolol (Corgard)	Slow the heart rate	Impotence, depression, may exacerbate asthma
ACE inhibitors	Captopril (Capoten) Lisinopril (Prinivil, Zestril) Enalapril (Vasotec) Ramipril (Altace) Perindropril (Aceon)	Block the production of angiotensin, a hormone that raises blood pressure	Persistent cough
Calcium channel blockers	Nifedipine (Procardia) Diltiazem (Cardizem) Verapamil (Calan, Isoptin) Amlodipine (Norvasc)	Relax the muscle cells that constrict the blood vessels	Leg swelling
Angiotensin receptor blockers	Losartan (Cozaar) Valsartan (Diovan) Candesartan (Atacand) Irbesartan (Avapro)	Block the effects of angiotensin, a hormone that raises blood pressure.	
Alpha blockers	Doxazosin (Cardura) Terazosin (Hytrin) Prazosin (Minipress)	Dilate the blood vessels	Orthostatic hypotension (excessive drop in blood pressure when standing up suddenly)
Centrally acting medications	Clonidine (Catapres)	Reduce blood pressure through control mechanisms in the brain	Depression

is an important problem but have considerable difficulty reducing her weight and risk, despite her best efforts. Modifiable risk factors can be further divided into "behavioral risks" and "medical risks."

BEHAVIORAL RISKS

Smoking. Smoking is a major preventable cause of stroke in the United States, second only to hypertension. Smoking is estimated to increase the risk of an ischemic stroke by 50 percent, and it also raises the risk of heart disease and cancer substantially. The more someone smokes, the greater that person's risk of having a stroke. Fortunately, this risk can be quickly lowered by discontinuing smoking. Even after fifty years of heavy smoking, an individual can reduce her risk of stroke immediately by quitting. Family members of a stroke survivor should also realize that "passive smoking" (inhaling someone else's tobacco smoke) is harmful as well and increases the risk of stroke significantly.

Diet. A diet rich in fruits, vegetables, and whole grains and low in fat can reduce the risk of stroke, as well as lower high blood pressure (an important medical risk factor discussed below). In the Framingham study, a long-term study of risk factors for stroke and heart disease, eating three servings of fruit or vegetables a day was associated with a 22 percent reduction in stroke risk. There are other benefits to this type of diet as well, including reducing the risk of other diseases (heart disease, colon cancer) and helping control weight. Finally, this type of diet is rich in vitamins such as folate, which may play a role in reducing the risk of stroke.

Physical activity. People who are physically active have a lower risk of stroke. In the Framingham study, moderate physical activity was found to reduce the risk of stroke by 60 percent. In another study, women who exercised had a 27 percent reduction in their risk of stroke. Interestingly, the type of physical activity doesn't seem to matter. The idea that intense exercise is needed to obtain these benefits is a common misconception. Even moderate levels of activity show significant advantages over a sedentary existence.

Many people with a history of stroke assume that they will be unable to exercise because of physical limitations such as weakness of the arm and leg. These challenges can be overcome, however, even in individuals who are substantially affected by their stroke. For individuals who are able, walking is an excellent form of exercise and serves to improve strength and coordination at the same time that it reduces the risk of another stroke. For individuals who require the use of a wheelchair, propelling the wheelchair can provide good exercise. Adapted use of exercise equipment, such as a recumbent bicycle (one in which the user sits) can also be an effective form of exercise for people with severe weakness after stroke. Motivation is a key factor in undertaking this type of exercise program, since it goes beyond the usual rehabilitation provided after stroke.

Previously sedentary individuals should not attempt to change their lifestyle in a single weekend. Gradual increases in exercise intensity and duration are clearly the best way to establish a regular exercise program. Anyone with a prior stroke should consult a physician before undertaking any program that includes moderate or high-intensity exercises.

Alcohol use. The relationship between alcohol use and stroke is a complex one. Whereas light use of alcohol (one drink a day) is associated with a reduced risk of ischemic stroke, alcohol use of any kind brings with it an increased risk of hemorrhagic stroke. The current consensus is that if someone doesn't already drink, he shouldn't start. If he already drinks lightly (and doesn't have a history of hemorrhagic stroke) it appears safe to continue. Even light alcohol use should be discussed with a physician, as certain medications or other medical circumstances may preclude any alcohol use after stroke. Moderate or heavy alcohol use is clearly hazardous after stroke and increases the risk of a hemorrhagic stroke, not to mention stomach and liver problems, as well as other adverse effects.

Obesity. Being significantly overweight increases the risk of stroke. This has been most clearly shown for women, but it is likely true for men as well. Being overweight can also contribute to the severity of diabetes and hypertension.

Controlling weight is difficult for many able-bodied people, and certainly no easier for people who have had a stroke. Research (and countless personal testimonies) has shown that it is very difficult to lose weight simply by reducing the amount eaten. The best approach is a combination of lifestyle changes, such as sharply reducing high-fat and sugary foods and substituting more fruits and vegetables, reducing the overall number of calories eaten, reducing in-between-meal snacks, and increasing exercise. Stroke survivors should be wary of "fad" diets, which can be risky and can sometimes affect important medical treatments such as Coumadin (warfarin) therapy.

MEDICAL RISK FACTORS

Hypertension. Elevated blood pressure has long been known to increase the risk of stroke, and it is the single largest preventable cause of stroke. The good news is that control of high blood pressure reduces this risk considerably. The ideal approach to blood pressure control should include lifestyle changes (such as exercise and a diet high in fruits and vegetables, which are both helpful in blood pressure reduction). If this is insufficient, many effective and well-tolerated medications exist to control hypertension.

Atrial fibrillation. Atrial fibrillation is well established as a risk factor for stroke, though the severity of this risk is somewhat dependent on other factors, such as age and other heart disease. Coumadin (warfarin) is the preferred treatment to prevent stroke for most people with this condition. Aspirin also has some benefit and is sometimes used if Coumadin cannot be given for medical reasons, and in selected individuals with a low risk of stroke.

Hyperlipidemia. Hyperlipidemia, or elevated blood cholesterol (and in particular, LDL cholesterol), is a risk factor for stroke as well as for heart disease. Diet plays an important role in hyperlipidemia. Indeed, a diet rich in fruits, vegetables, and whole grains and low in saturated fats can help lower cholesterol. If diet alone is insufficient, treatment with the cholesterol-lowering drugs known as statins can reduce the risk of stroke significantly.

Diabetes. Diabetes is a known risk factor for stroke. As with hypertension, the degree of risk is reduced if this condition is well controlled. Achieving good control of diabetes requires more than just the right combination of medicines. Careful attention to diet, increasing exercise, and controlling weight are all very important in controlling diabetes. In many cases, these nonmedical approaches can also reduce the need for medication or insulin. Good control of hypertension is particularly important for stroke prevention in people with diabetes.

Carotid stenosis. Narrowing of either of the carotid arteries, the major blood vessels on each side of the neck, increases the risk of stroke. The degree of risk depends in part on the severity of the narrowing. Many of these blockages develop gradually and may be asymptomatic. Surgery has been shown to reduce the risk of future stroke in individuals with moderate to severe narrowing ("stenosis") of these blood vessels, particularly those who have had related symptoms, such as a TIA.

Homocysteine. Homocysteine is a substance that is normally found in blood. In the last few years, elevated levels of homocysteine have been found to be associated with a higher risk of stroke. Homocysteine levels can be lowered with supplementary vitamins (folate, vitamins B6 and B12). While many physicians suspect that lowering homocysteine through the use of vitamins will reduce the risk of stroke, this has not yet been proven in definitive research studies. Some physicians are advising patients at risk for a stroke to take daily vitamin supplements as they await final results from ongoing research studies.

C-reactive protein. C-reactive protein (CRP) is a chemical in the blood that provides information about ongoing, low-level inflammation. Recent research has demonstrated that measurement of this protein helps predict a person's risk of cardiovascular disease, including stroke. This test is not yet widely used, and active debate continues within the medical community regarding when and for whom CRP should be measured. Although treatments to specifically lower CRP are not yet available, identifying people at increased risk may help target other treatments, such as the use of statin medications.

Nonmodifiable Risk Factors

Some of the risk factors for stroke can't be changed. These include age, sex, racial/ethnic background, history of prior stroke, and family history.

Although these risk factors can't be modified, they are important to understand and may provide people with an impetus to work harder on some of the modifiable risk factors discussed above.

AGE

Like many diseases, the risk of stroke rises as people age. This increase is gradual until age fifty, after which the risk of stroke doubles each decade.

SEX

Men have a slightly higher risk of stroke than women.

RACE/ETHNICITY

Certain racial and ethnic groups have higher risk of stroke than other groups. For example, the risk of stroke in African-Americans is estimated to be 38 percent higher than in white Americans. The reasons underlying these racial and ethnic differences remain controversial and may in fact represent a combination of environmental influences and genetic factors.

FAMILY HISTORY

People with a family history of stroke have a higher risk of stroke than the general population.

The fact that someone may have one or more nonmodifiable stroke risk factors shouldn't lead to a sense of futility or fatalism regarding stroke. To the contrary, these nonmodifiable risk factors can be viewed as a "call to action" to more aggressively reduce the impact of other, modifiable risk factors.

Jim is a sixty-four-year-old man who has recently developed TIAs. He is now taking aspirin to reduce his risk of another stroke but wants to do as much as possible in the way of prevention. He consults his physician, who notes that Jim frequently forgets to take his medication for high blood pressure. They agree that Jim will try a once-a-day medication to make it easier for him to remember to take his medication consistently. Jim agrees to stop smoking and begins using a nicotine patch and attending a smoking-cessation support group to help him with this important lifestyle change. He agrees to begin a gradual exercise program with his wife, focusing on walking each day. Jim and his wife decide to stop eating at fast-food restaurants and reduce the amount of high-fat food in their diets to help lower cholesterol and assist with weight control. Six months later, Jim has lost fifteen pounds (and his wife is pleased that she has lost ten pounds as well!), has not resumed smoking, and is feeling more fit than he has in twenty years. When following up with his physician, Jim says, "You know, that TIA may have been the best thing that ever happened to me. It forced me to clean up my act."

Prevention of Hemorrhagic Stroke

Prevention for hemorrhagic stroke differs from prevention for ischemic stroke, though some aspects are similar.

Medications

A number of medications can cause or contribute to a cerebral hemorrhage. Coumadin (warfarin) can cause cerebral hemorrhage, most typically if the dosage is too high for a particular individual and the anticoagulant effects too pronounced (this can be checked by use of the INR test). Aspirin can also be a contributing cause, though it is not sufficient by itself to cause a hemorrhage in an otherwise healthy person. Other anti-inflammatory medications, such as ibuprofen (Motrin, Advil) or naproxen (Aleve), can also contribute to a tendency to bleed and should not be used by anyone who has had a prior cerebral hemorrhage or is at risk for one (for example, if the person has a known AVM) unless discussed with a physician.

Hypertension

Hypertension (elevated blood pressure) is a major risk factor for hemorrhagic stroke. Effective control of blood pressure is one of the most important preventive measures for hemorrhagic stroke.

Alcohol

Alcohol usage is clearly associated with an increased risk of cerebral hemorrhage. Some physicians allow patients with a history of a prior hemorrhage to have an occasional drink, though I advise my patients against drinking altogether.

Smoking

Smoking has long been known to be a risk factor for ischemic stroke, but recently it has been identified as a risk factor for hemorrhagic stroke as well. Smoking cessation is an important aspect of preventing a recurrent hemorrhagic stroke.

4

How the Brain Works

Michelle is a seventy-three-year-old woman who experiences a brief episode during which she is unable to speak. The episode lasts for approximately ten minutes and has completely resolved by the time she is evaluated by her physician. She is diagnosed with a transient ischemic attack (TIA). Her evaluation for the TIA includes an MRI scan of the brain. She is shocked when the MRI scan shows an old small stroke in an area of the brain that is completely unrelated to her TIA symptoms. She asks her physician, "How could I have had a stroke and not had any symptoms?"

Frank develops sudden and severe weakness on his right side. His MRI shows a lacunar stroke in the part of the brain known as the pons. When discussing with Frank the results of his MRI scan, his physician notes that it was a very small stroke. Frank questions her, "Why did such a small stroke cause such severe symptoms?"

The relationship between the size and location of a stroke and the symptoms it produces is complicated. As a general rule, however, the location of a stroke is more important than its size in determining the severity of the symptoms. A small stroke that occurs in a very vital area can cause severe symptoms. A stroke of the same size in another area of the brain might not even be noticed by the affected person. In fact, it is quite common for individuals with a "first" stroke to have evidence of prior "silent" small strokes on their CT or MRI scans.

What follows is a general introduction to the anatomy of the brain.

Each of the symptoms caused by strokes in these various parts of the brain is discussed in further detail in subsequent chapters.

The brain is an incredibly complex biological computer that can accomplish feats far beyond the capabilities of the most sophisticated computers Silicon Valley can produce. Owing to its complexity, there is still much that we do not know about how the human brain processes information, creates thoughts and feelings, and produces consciousness and self-awareness. Much of what we do know about the brain's functions has come from careful study of people who have had strokes. By comparing the location of the damage in the brain to the lost function, physicians have gradually learned about the function of each area of the brain.

The brain processes information through a complex and highly interconnected network of cells known as neurons. It is estimated that there are more than 100 billion neurons in the adult brain. These cells are responsible for the major work of the brain. Unlike most desktop computers, which have only one main processor of information, each of the brain's neurons can be considered a simple computer. When connected together, these billions of cells create a very sophisticated biological computer. The fact that each neuron in the brain can process information independently allows the brain to work on multiple tasks at once. For example, the healthy brain can control the chewing and swallowing of popcorn while simultaneously watching a movie.

Neurons are connected to each other through a network of filamentous structures known as axons and dendrites, which transmit electrical impulses like wires. At the actual site of the connection to other neurons are specialized links known as synapses. The end of the nerve axon (known as the nerve terminal) releases specialized chemicals into the space between it and the adjacent neuron. These chemicals, known as neurotransmitters, then cause a reaction in the adjacent neuron. In the right circumstances, the second neuron then relays an electrical impulse through its own axons to the other neurons to which it is connected. In a sense, these transmissions are almost like a game of telephone, whereby each neuron passes along the message to the next. As in the game of telephone, however, the message changes as it moves along. Imagine a person stepping on a sharp object. The nerve cells pick up the message in the foot and relay it to a neuron in the part of the brain that feels pain.

These neurons send a message to the part of the brain that regulates movement. The neurons then direct a message to the muscles in the leg to move the foot away from the sharp object.

In addition to the neurons that perform the actual computation, the brain contains many other cells and structures that provide support for the neurons. These include the cells known as glia, which perform a variety of functions, including providing an insulating layer for the axons and dendrites, providing structural support, and helping to fight off infection.

The brain consumes a lot of energy processing all the information that comes to it. In fact, about 25 percent of the body's energy usage occurs in the brain. As a result, the brain is very dependent on a steady supply of blood to bring it the fuel it needs to carry out its functions. This fuel consists primarily of sugar (glucose), as well as the oxygen the brain needs to "burn" this fuel.

The brain is a very soft and fragile organ with a consistency often compared to Jell-O. For this reason, the body has evolved a protective system around the brain to prevent it from being injured. A special clear fluid known as cerebrospinal fluid surrounds the brain and provides a liquid cushion around it. The brain also has a tough membrane, known as the dura, surrounding it to provide further protection. Lastly, it is encased in a very strong, hard case made of bone—the skull.

The brain does not function as a single, undifferentiated organ. Rather, it has a variety of specialized structures and functions. Each area of the brain is associated with specific functions. Given the complexity of the human brain, it is not surprising that these functions are closely interrelated between different areas. For this reason, multiple areas of the brain often participate in complex functions such as movement, sensation, speech, and thinking abilities.

Crossed Controls

Control of movement and sensation is primarily located in the opposite side of the brain from the body part. Thus movements of the left hand are primarily controlled by the right side of the brain, and vice versa. Similarly, if the left hand is touched, the sensation is transmitted to the right side of the brain. Visual information processing follows a similar design, with images of objects on a person's left side processed by the right side of the brain.

One exception to this general rule of crossed controls involves the cerebellum, the right side of which helps controls the right side of the body. Another exception consists of certain cranial nerve control centers in the brainstem that are on the same side of the brain as the area of the body controlled.

Right vs. Left Brain: Are They Different?

The brain is a fairly symmetrical organ, with the right and left halves having nearly identical mirror-image structures. While the two sides of the brain may look the same, certain functions, such as language, are based more on one side than the other. Since language is so important, the side of the brain that provides this function is known as the "dominant" side. This is usually the left side of the brain.

Most people are right-handed and have left cerebral dominance, that is, language is based on the left side of their brains. Even most left-handed people have a similar pattern of cerebral dominance. In a few individuals, however (most commonly left-handed), there is a reversed pattern of cerebral dominance, and language is based on the right side instead of the left. Many of these individuals have some degree of mixed dominance, wherein the division of labor between the two sides of the brain is less distinct than usual. Right or mixed cerebral dominance does not cause any symptoms and only becomes evident when a stroke occurs.

There are extensive connections between the two sides of the brain to ensure that they remain well coordinated. In a few cases of stroke, these connections are sufficiently damaged so that the left hand literally doesn't know what the right hand is doing. This condition is known as the "alien hand" syndrome and can be quite distressing to the person experiencing it. In this condition, the hand (usually the left) seems to act on its own accord. In reality, the right side of the brain is not receiving sufficient information from the left side, and thus may generate movements that don't make sense to the left side of the brain. Treatments are still being studied and include methods to try to make the right side of the brain more aware of the dominant left side's intentions.

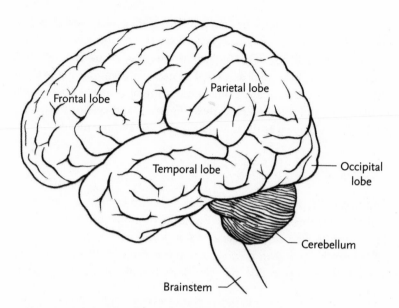

FIGURE 4.1   *Major areas of the brain (surface view).*
This side view of the brain shows the major lobes of the cerebral cortex,
including frontal lobe, parietal lobe, occipital lobe, and temporal lobe, as well
as the cerebellum and brainstem.

Major Parts of the Brain

The brain has several major structures, each of which has a variety of distinct subparts and functions (see Figure 4.1).

Brainstem

The most basic part of the brain is the lowest part, known as the brainstem. This is the part of the brain that evolved first. It controls basic functions such as breathing and wakefulness. It is also the conduit through which virtually all other brain activities funnel on their way to the rest of the body. This part of the brain is not involved directly in thinking, though if damaged sufficiently, it fails to keep awake the portions of the brain where thinking occurs. In the most severe cases, damage to the brainstem can cause coma or even death. In other cases, brainstem damage can cause severe weakness, loss of sensation, and swallowing difficulties. The small size of the brainstem and its tightly packed structures make it vulnerable to small areas of damage. A small stroke in the brainstem can cause much more pronounced symptoms than a larger stroke in many areas of the cerebral cortex. The brainstem contains three distinct sections, known as the midbrain, the pons, and the medulla.

Cerebellum

Attached to the brainstem is a sizable structure known as the cerebellum. The cerebellum plays a key role in coordination of movement. Damage to this area can cause a loss of coordination, known as ataxia. The cerebellum's role in thinking remains controversial, with some evidence that damage in this area can impact thinking abilities in subtle ways.

Thalamus

Perched on top of the brainstem is the thalamus, which plays a critical role in the brain as a kind of relay station. The thalamus has connections to many different areas of the brain, and damage in this area can cause a wide range of problems. Damage to the sensory relays in the thalamus can cause severe sensory loss and pain problems. Thalamic damage can affect motivation and initiative through its connections to the frontal lobes. Language can also be affected by thalamic injury.

Cerebral Cortex

Finally, wrapped around the thalamus is the cerebral cortex. This is a wrinkled-looking structure that forms the surface of the brain. The cerebral cortex is where the most sophisticated brain functions reside. The cerebral cortex consists of two halves, or hemispheres (right and left). Each hemisphere is commonly divided into several major sections, known as lobes, on the basis of each lobe's structure and functions.

FRONTAL LOBE

The frontal lobe is, as its name implies, at the front of the brain, behind the eyes. The frontal lobe is responsible for modulating behavior and setting priorities. Damage to this area can cause a variety of behavioral and personality changes, such as loss of initiative, uninhibited behavior, or inability to focus on appropriate activities. The portion of the frontal lobe that borders on the parietal lobe (see below) is known as the motor cortex. This strip of brain tissue is the primary controller for movement on the opposite side of the body. Injuries to this area of the brain can cause weakness and loss of coordination.

A portion of the frontal lobe at the lower end of the motor strip is known as Broca's area. This area controls speech production. Damage to this area can cause difficulty in expressing thoughts through language (nonfluent aphasia).

THE PARIETAL LOBE

The parietal lobe sits directly behind the frontal lobe. The part that is adjacent to the frontal lobe is known as the primary sensory cortex. This area provides a major portion of the brain's ability to perceive sensations coming from the opposite side of the body. Damage to this area can cause numbness of the opposite side of the body.

The parietal lobes are also responsible for self-awareness of the body. Damage to the parietal lobe (particularly the right parietal lobe) can result in difficulty recognizing parts of one's own body and difficulty determining the body's orientation in space.

The area of the parietal lobe behind the sensory cortex is responsible for making logical connections and processing information. Mathematical ability, understanding of time and sequence, memories of how to perform familiar activities, and aspects of language are all functions of the parietal lobes.

THE OCCIPITAL LOBE

The occipital lobe sits at the back of the brain, immediately behind the parietal lobe. The occipital lobe processes the information from the eyes and is responsible for visual perception. Damage to this area can cause loss of visual perception and partial or even complete blindness.

THE TEMPORAL LOBE

The temporal lobe curves forward from the occipital lobe and the lower portion of the parietal lobes. The temporal lobe plays a key role in the storage of long-term memories. Fortunately, the body seems to share the storage of these memories between the two sides of the brain, so injuries to this area on one side as a result of stroke do not usually cause severe loss of long-term memory. Damage to both sides, however, can be devastating.

The portion of the temporal lobe (usually the left) adjacent to the parietal lobe is known as Wernicke's area and is responsible for language comprehension. Damage to this area can cause a fluent aphasia as well as the inability to understand language.

THE LIMBIC SYSTEM

The limbic system consists of structures on the "inside" surface of the brain—that is, facing directly toward the other hemisphere of the brain. The limbic system plays a key role in regulating basic emotions, such as fear, aggression, and sexual urges.

The Motor and Sensory Maps

As noted, the frontal and parietal lobes contain the primary motor-control area and the primary sensory-perception area, respectively. These areas are arranged in a very specific fashion, with control of parts of the body consistently located in the same portion of these strips (see Figure 4.2). These "maps" of the brain's organization are often referred to as the motor and the sensory "homunculus." Although all areas of the body are represented in these structures, the relative amount of brain tissue devoted to each area is proportional to the functional demands of each area rather than to its size. Thus the lips, tongue, and fingers have very large representations in these structures owing to the fine degree of motor control and sensory ability that these areas require. Large areas such as the torso have relatively small representation. The relationship between these maps and the blood supply to the brain is responsible for some of

Motor (precentral gyrus)

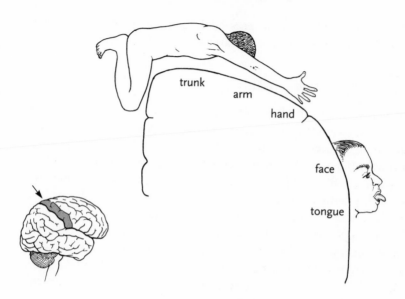

Sensory (postcentral gyrus)

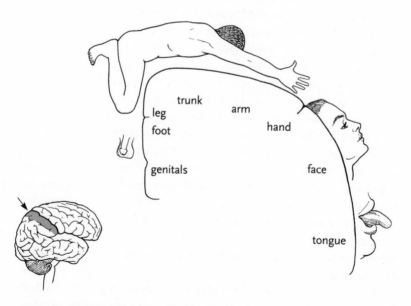

FIGURE 4.2   *Map of the primary motor and sensory control areas of the brain.*

the common patterns of weakness and sensory loss seen with blockage
of the middle or anterior cerebral arteries.

Blood Supply to the Brain

The brain receives its blood supply from three main blood vessels (arteries): the two carotid arteries (one on each side of the neck) and the basilar
artery in the back of the neck and brainstem (see Figure 4.3). These
main arteries each split up into several branches, similar to a tree. These
branches, in turn, progressively split into smaller and smaller branches,
until they become the smallest blood vessels, known as capillaries. The
capillaries have very thin walls and allow the nutrients and oxygen in the
blood both to pass through the blood vessel walls into the adjacent cells
in the brain and to absorb the waste products of these same cells. The
capillaries then drain into tiny veins to carry blood back toward the heart.
These veins progressively join together to form larger veins that carry the
blood into the neck and beyond.

Ischemic strokes are caused by blockage of blood vessels (virtually always arteries, though blocked veins can also cause stroke on occasion).
The larger the blood vessel that is blocked, the larger the area of the brain
that is deprived of its blood supply, and the larger the resulting stroke.
Thus blockages of a carotid artery may cause a very large stroke; blockage
of one of the smaller branches deep within the brain would cause a small
stroke. Because of the brain's exceptional importance, coupled with its
sensitivity to interruption of blood flow, the human brain has evolved
somewhat of a backup system for these main arteries. This system is
known as the "Circle of Willis" (see Figure 4.4). This circle (really more of
a polygon) consists of small arteries around the base of the brain that
connect the two carotid arteries with each other and the basilar artery. Because of this system, some people can have a severe injury or complete
blockage of one of the main arteries in the neck but not experience any
symptoms. In such cases the other arteries are able to supply the areas
beyond the blockage through the Circle of Willis, and maintain sufficient
blood supply to the brain.

Unfortunately, the Circle of Willis is not always complete and fully
functioning. Some people are born missing one of the small connecting
arteries or may experience a blockage of these arteries. Others have a

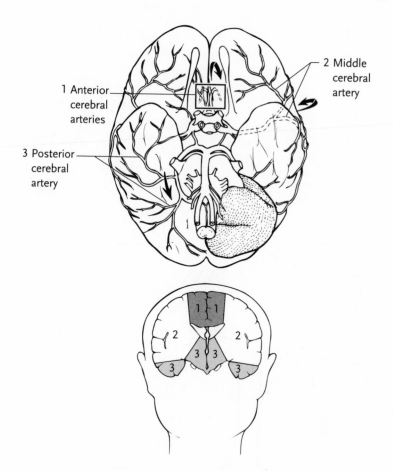

1 Anterior cerebral arteries

2 Middle cerebral artery

3 Posterior cerebral artery

FIGURE 4.3   *Vascular supply of the brain.*
Shown here are the major arteries supplying blood to the brain, as well as the areas supplied by these arteries.

complete circle but the connecting arteries are too small to carry enough blood to compensate for a blockage of one of the main arteries. Furthermore, many strokes also occur downstream from the Circle of Willis, where no comparable backup system exists.

Blockage of each of the main arteries of the brain causes a distinct pattern of damage to the brain. Despite some variation from person to per-

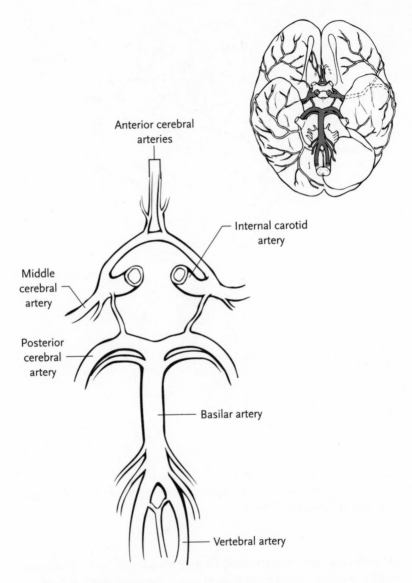

FIGURE 4.4 *Circle of Willis.*
This diagram shows the blood vessels at the base of the brain that form the
Circle of Willis.

son in the blood supply to the brain and in the location of various brain functions, generally the location of a blockage in a major artery to the brain causes a fairly predictable set of symptoms for the stroke survivor. These patterns are known as stroke syndromes. Some of the more common syndromes are described below (a full description of all syndromes is beyond the scope of this book).

Middle Cerebral Artery Stroke

Middle cerebral artery strokes typically affect portions of the frontal lobe, parietal lobe, and temporal lobe. Severe weakness of the affected side is common, and the leg is often somewhat less affected than the arm. Aphasia occurs with left middle cerebral artery strokes, and cognitive problems with right-sided strokes. Visual loss to the affected side is common as well.

Middle Cerebral Artery: Inferior vs. Superior Division Strokes

The middle cerebral artery generally divides into two major parts—the inferior (lower) and the superior (upper). Strokes may affect just one of these two divisions. Strokes affecting the superior division generally cause weakness but less language or cognitive disturbance. Inferior-division strokes typically cause language difficulties (if affecting the left side) or cognitive difficulties (if affecting the right side), but tend not to cause weakness. Loss of vision to the affected side is another common feature of inferior-division strokes.

Anterior Cerebral Artery Stroke

The anterior cerebral artery supplies blood to large portions of the frontal lobe. A stroke affecting this artery may cause frontal lobe cognitive symptoms, such as loss of initiative, as well as weakness that affects the leg but not the hand.

Carotid Occlusion

Blockage of the carotid artery can cause combined middle cerebral artery and anterior cerebral artery strokes on the same side of the brain. Severe weakness of the affected side is usual. Strokes affecting the left side of the brain will commonly cause severe (global) aphasia. Those on the right side of the brain will result in left neglect (loss of awareness of the left side) and other cognitive symptoms (see Chapter 13).

Posterior Cerebral Artery Stroke

Strokes affecting the posterior cerebral artery cause visual loss as a result of damage to the occipital lobe. They also commonly cause a visual neglect (reduced attention to the affected side). Memory difficulties may result, especially if both sides are affected.

Internal Capsular Stroke

Internal capsular strokes are usually smaller strokes and cause primarily weakness, loss of sensation, or both.

Pontine Stroke

Small strokes in the pons (a portion of the brainstem) commonly cause weakness of the affected side. Larger strokes in the pons can sometimes cause severe weakness of both sides, resulting in a condition known as the "Locked-in syndrome," in which movement is lost in all four limbs, and the only remaining movements are certain eye movements.

Lateral Medullary Stroke (Wallenberg Syndrome)

A stroke in the medulla (a portion of the brainstem) can cause a combination of severe swallowing difficulties, dizziness, loss of balance and coordination, and loss of sensation.

Cerebellar Strokes

Strokes affecting the cerebellum can result in loss of balance and coordination. These strokes often affect areas of the brainstem as well, with resulting sensory loss and/or weakness. A combination of weakness on one side and ataxia (loss of coordination) on the other side is possible.

Locations of Brain Hemorrhage

As with ischemic stroke, there are certain common patterns for cerebral hemorrhage, which tends to affect certain areas of the brain preferentially.

Frontal Hemorrhage

Hemorrhage in the frontal area of the brain commonly causes reduced initiative. Weakness is usually absent or mild.

Basal Ganglia Hemorrhage

Basal ganglia hemorrhages typically cause symptoms similar to those seen in middle cerebral artery strokes, including weakness, loss of sensation, language (left-side) or cognitive (right-side) difficulties.

Occipital Hemorrhage

Hemorrhage in the occipital area usually results in visual loss to the affected side.

Thalamic Hemorrhage

The symptoms resulting from thalamic hemorrhage vary with location. Loss of sensation, which may be quite severe, is a common result of thalamic hemorrhage. Large hemorrhages in the thalamus can lead to lethargy and loss of initiative.

Cerebellar Hemorrhage

Cerebellar hemorrhage generally causes loss of coordination (ataxia).

Anterior Communicating Aneurysm Rupture

The anterior communicating artery is a common location for aneurysms. When aneurysms rupture, loss of initiation and attention problems often result.

Other Important Neurological Structures

Spinal Cord

The brain connects with most of the rest of the body through the brainstem and on through the spinal cord. The spinal cord serves as a conduit for information to and from the brain from the trunk and limbs. Damage to the spinal cord is often due to trauma, though it can also occur after a loss of blood supply (similar to a stroke affecting the brain), bleeding, or tumors. Damage to the spinal cord can cause weakness, sensory loss, or complete paralysis.

Peripheral Nerves

The peripheral nerves connect the spinal cord to the skin, muscles, and other internal structures. These are the wires of the body, bringing information to and from the spinal cord, where it is ultimately transmitted to the brain. Damage to the nerves can occur in many conditions, most notably diabetes. Stroke does not directly affect the functioning of the nerves, but rather affects the processing of the information obtained through these nerves, and the creation of messages to the muscles sent via the nerves.

Cranial Nerves

The nerves to the head and neck largely bypass the spinal cord and have direct connections to the brain. There are twelve pairs of specialized nerves that connect directly to the brain, known as the cranial nerves. In addition to providing control of muscles and the usual senses of touch, these nerves also provide several special senses. These include vision, hearing, balance (vestibular), taste, and smell. The cranial nerves are essential for swallowing, since they provide control of the tongue and swallowing muscles. The control centers for most of the cranial nerves are located in the brainstem, and damage to this area can severely affect the functioning of these nerves. For this reason, brainstem strokes can cause severe loss of sensation and/or weakness of the face, eye movements, and severe difficulty swallowing.

Measuring the Function of the Brain

New techniques now allow us to record the functioning of the brain directly. These include imaging techniques, such as functional MRI (fMRI), positron emission tomography (PET) scanning, magnetoencephalography, and near-infrared spectroscopy, which provide pictures of brain functioning. Other techniques, such as transcortical magnetic stimulation, evoked potentials, and electroencephalography (EEG), are used to measure the functioning of the brain without creating images, These methods have not yet entered routine clinical practice for stroke but are used as research tools. With these new techniques we are gaining insights into the relationship between brain structure, function, and the effects of stroke that will ultimately influence stroke treatment and rehabilitation.

Medical Complications after Stroke

Ron is a seventy-four-year-old man admitted to the county hospital after suddenly losing the ability to speak and developing severe right-sided weakness. Shortly after admission it becomes clear that he is not able to pass his urine, and a Foley catheter (a thin rubber tube) is placed in his bladder to drain the urine. His blood pressure is markedly elevated on arrival to the hospital, and he requires multiple new medications to control it. As a result of difficulty swallowing, he develops pneumonia three days after admission and requires intravenous antibiotics. When he is transferred to a rehabilitation hospital after nine days in the county hospital, he is found to have both a urinary infection and a blood clot in his leg. He is placed on an oral antibiotic for the urinary infection and is given Fragmin (dalteparin) and subsequently Coumadin (warfarin) for the blood clot. The Foley (urinary) catheter is removed, but he has difficulty passing his urine. Ultimately, the urologist feels that an enlarged prostate is contributing to his difficulty voiding, and he is placed on tamsulosin (Flomax), with improved ability to empty his bladder. His blood pressure in the rehabilitation hospital is mildly elevated, but doctors feel no change in his blood pressure medication is necessary. His family is concerned by Ron's multiple medical complications. Is this "normal" after a stroke? Will his medical condition stabilize over time?

Ron's case is not unusual. Stroke is often complicated by medical problems that are related to the stroke but require recognition and specific treatment. Medical complications can occur early or late after stroke, and the types of problems that develop vary over time. Some of these are preventable with good medical care, whereas others are unavoidable.

Early complications frequently include pneumonia, urinary infections, and urinary retention (inability to pass urine). Later complications can include osteoporosis and urinary frequency. This chapter provides an overview of some of the most common medical issues that occur after stroke.

Hypertension

Hypertension (elevated blood pressure) is an important risk factor for stroke, as well as a medical issue frequently requiring attention afterward. In some cases, blood pressure temporarily increases at the time of the stroke but then gradually returns to its normal level. Although elevated blood pressure is an important risk factor for stroke, it is important not to reduce blood pressure too quickly or too severely immediately after a stroke, since this may actually worsen the effects of the stroke. Lowering the blood pressure too abruptly after a stroke may reduce blood supply to areas receiving a marginal supply as a result of a blocked or partially blocked blood vessel. Some centers are actually studying medications to elevate blood pressure temporarily at the time of an acute stroke in carefully selected individuals, though this is not a standard treatment.

Opinions vary, but many neurologists recommend allowing mild hypertension during the first few weeks after a stroke, and then gradually bringing blood pressure under tighter control. In the long run, controlling hypertension remains a very important method of reducing the risk of another stroke.

Diabetes

Diabetes is a risk factor for stroke and thus very common among stroke survivors. Some research suggests that controlling elevated blood sugars may help reduce the extent of neurological damage at the time of a stroke. The body's response to the physical stress of stroke often includes a temporary elevation in blood sugar levels in diabetics. After a stroke, the combination of medical illness, lack of usual activity levels, and changes in diet often adversely affects the control of diabetes. These factors may continue to do so for some time after stroke, and many individuals return home receiving significantly different diabetes treatment programs than before the stroke. It is important for family members to participate in the monitoring of blood sugars after return home, as the dose of oral medication or insulin required will likely change significantly once the patient is released from the hospital.

Bladder Problems

Stroke often affects bladder function, though the issues can be quite different early after stroke compared with later. Soon after a stroke it is quite common for the patient to experience urinary retention—an inability to pass urine even when the bladder is full. Urinary retention after stroke may be caused by a temporary weakness of the muscles in the bladder that normally contract to squeeze the urine out. This weakness can be a direct symptom of the stroke, or can sometimes result from an "overstretch" injury to the bladder. In overstretch injury, the bladder nerves and muscles are damaged by a severely distended bladder that is not emptied promptly. This can occur in a person who collapses from a stroke and is not discovered for a lengthy period, or even in someone who is receiving medical attention but is too confused from the stroke to empty his bladder.

Bladder function may also be affected by other, nonstroke problems that may first become evident after a stroke. The most common of these are benign prostatic hypertrophy (BPH) in men and stress incontinence in women. Careful evaluation of bladder symptoms by a physician should distinguish among these possibilities.

Urinary retention is usually treated with the temporary placement of a Foley catheter in the bladder. While this provides an immediate short-term solution to the problem of urinary retention, these catheters can lead to infections and so should be removed as soon as possible. In some cases, urinary function recovers quickly and normal urination resumes once the catheter is removed. In other cases, however, the recovery is more prolonged. When this happens, many rehabilitation facilities will switch to a treatment known as "intermittent catheterization," in which a urinary catheter is placed into the bladder several times a day to empty the bladder, and then immediately removed. This allows the bladder to gradually regain its normal function over time, and actually has a lower risk of infection than leaving the catheter in place.

Urinary incontinence is the inability to control the emptying of the bladder. This problem is very common early after a stroke and may have several causes. The most serious cause is a condition known as "overflow" incontinence. As the name implies, this type of incontinence is caused by a full bladder literally overflowing with urine. This form of urinary retention needs to be identified promptly so that appropriate treatment (generally catheterization) can be instituted. In many rehabilitation facilities, this condition can be easily and non-invasively assessed by a nurse using a simple ultrasound device at the bedside known as a Bladderscan. This device can measure the amount of urine present in the bladder and determine if there is urinary retention. An alternative technique involves placing a catheter in the bladder after voiding to determine how much urine remains in the bladder.

In most cases of urinary incontinence after stroke, retention is not the cause. Often several factors combine to cause incontinence. For many individuals, cognitive or communication issues may impede their ability to control their bladder. A person with aphasia after a stroke may be unable to let her nurse know that she needs to urinate. Someone who is confused after a stroke may not recognize the sensation of needing to empty his bladder or understand the use of the call bell. These cognitive and communication issues are often more severe at night, and nocturnal incontinence is particularly common after stroke.

Other factors contributing to urinary incontinence may be urinary infections or an overactive detrussor muscle (see "Frequent Urination" below). Lastly, many stroke survivors are unable to get to the bathroom safely by themselves early on after a stroke, and so are dependent on the timely assistance of nursing staff. Delays in obtaining nursing assistance in a hospital or skilled nursing facility can be major contributors to incontinence.

In most cases, urinary incontinence improves over a period of weeks as cognitive and communication abilities and physical mobility improve. Many individuals experience improvements in continence after returning home, where caregivers are more consistently attuned to their bladder-management needs. Frequent scheduled trips to the bathroom (for example, every two hours) can help manage urinary incontinence by providing an opportunity to empty the bladder before it fills up and the urge to urinate occurs. This strategy of scheduled bathroom trips can be very effective in a hospital or nursing home environment or at home.

It is important to recognize that severe constipation can contribute to bladder malfunction, and treatment of the constipation may help restore more normal bladder function. Gravity and positioning play an important role in bladder emptying. Many individuals find urinating in a bedpan while lying on their back difficult or impossible. Sitting on a commode, or using a urinal while sitting at the edge of the bed, can make the difference between urinating normally and requiring a catheter.

Urine Infections

Urine infections are very common after stroke, particularly in the hospital or nursing home setting. These are caused by multiple factors. The use of catheters (particularly indwelling Foley catheters) allows bacteria access into the bladder. Difficulty emptying the bladder causes the urine to stagnate and any bacteria more time to establish an infection. Inadequate fluid intake is common after stroke, causing stagnation of urine owing to reduced frequency of bladder emptying. Preventive treatment includes removing urinary catheters as soon as possible, converting indwelling catheters to intermittent catheterization, and maintaining adequate fluid intake. Urinary infections are usually treated with oral antibiotics, though in severe cases intravenous antibiotics may be needed.

Frequent Urination

In the weeks to months after a stroke, the most common long-term bladder problem is excessively frequent urination. This is often accompanied by difficulty holding back the urge to urinate when it occurs. A patient with these symptoms should be tested for a urinary infection, since these are common symptoms for that condition. This is particularly important if the patient experiences an abrupt onset of symptoms or an abrupt change in symptoms. In most cases, however, persistent urinary frequency after a stroke is due to a reduction in control of the primary muscle controlling the bladder, known as the detrussor muscle. After a stroke the detrusor muscle may become "overactive" and begin emptying the bladder even when the bladder is not very full. Furthermore, the patient's control over the muscle is reduced, so it becomes harder to inhibit the activity of this overactive muscle. Certain medications, known as anticholinergic medications, are helpful in reducing the activity of this muscle. Some of the more common medications used for this purpose include tolterodine (Detrol), hyoscyamine (Cystospaz), and oxybutynin (Ditropan). All these medications share certain side effects, including dry mouth, urinary retention, and occasionally confusion in the elderly. By starting at a low dose and monitoring for side effects, most patients can usually tolerate these medications well.

It is important to recognize that some medications may actually worsen bladder problems after a stroke. Diuretics, also known as "water pills," are medications used to control high blood pressure or remove excess fluid. These include furosemide (Lasix), bumetanide (Bumex), hydrochlorthiazide, and others. Since these medications increase the amount of urine produced, they may contribute to the urgent need to empty the bladder and lead to incontinence. Sleeping medications such as zolpidem (Ambien), oxazepam (Serax), and many others can also contribute to urinary incontinence. By causing people to sleep more deeply, these drugs increase the likelihood that people will fail to respond to their bodies' needs, particularly at night. For this and other reasons, these medications should be used sparingly if not avoided altogether after stroke.

Bowel Problems

Bowel function is frequently affected by a stroke, though it usually returns to normal over time. The most common bowel symptom after stroke is constipation, which usually results from a combination of factors, including immobility, inadequate fluid intake, change in diet (with inadequate dietary fiber), change in bowel habits, and, in some cases, cognitive and communication issues. The preferred treatment is to resume a well-balanced diet with sufficient dietary fiber (contained in fruits, vegetables, and whole grains) and fluid intake. If this does not solve the problem or is not feasible (for example, because of swallowing difficulties), the next step is medical treatment, which in the hospital or nursing home generally consists of stool softeners such as docusate (Colace), bowel stimulants (Senna, Dulcolax), and/or laxatives (milk of magnesia, lactulose syrup, magnesium citrate). The use of fiber supplements (Metamucil, Citrucel) may be helpful in some cases, though these need to be combined with adequate fluid intake, or they may actually worsen constipation symptoms. Enemas are generally best avoided, though they are occasionally helpful as a one-time treatment in severe constipation. The restoration of physical mobility (for example, getting out of bed and walking) is an important factor in the eventual resolution of constipation. Developing a bowel "routine" can be helpful, with the use of bowel stimulants in combination with bowel evacuation at a standard time (say, after breakfast each day) often a key step in restoring more consistent bowel function.

Diarrhea or loose bowels are less common after stroke but do occur. In some cases, loose bowel movements can represent oozing of stool around a partial blockage due to severe constipation. A rectal examination by the nurse or physician can determine if this is responsible. In other cases, loose bowels are due to the use of antibiotics for an unrelated condition, such as a urinary infection or pneumonia. Some cases of antibiotic-related diarrhea are caused by a proliferation of abnormal bacteria in the large intestine known as "Clostridium Difficile," sometimes called "C-Diff." This can be a serious condition, and stool testing is widely available to check for it. Ironically, though this condition is caused by antibiotics, its treatment also involves antibiotics. The usual treatment is oral metronidazole (Flagyl), with vancomycin used in refractory cases. Loose bowel movements can sometimes result from excessive use of bowel medications, or from an intolerance to a nutritional formula used for tube feeding.

Bowel incontinence is less common after stroke than bladder incontinence, but it can occur in some cases. Similar factors are often involved, including alterations in communication and cognition. Adopting a bowel routine is often the most effective approach.

Seizures

Seizures are uncontrolled electrical activity in the brain that commonly result in loss of consciousness and uncontrolled movements (convulsions). While most people who have had a stroke will never have a seizure, seizures do affect approximately 10 percent of stroke survivors. Seizures may be one of the first symptoms of a stroke, or can first occur months or years after a stroke. The damage to the brain from a stroke can cause a "scar" to form in the brain, which then becomes a location for the seizure to start. Once a seizure is under way, it often spreads through the brain. When the seizure affects only part of the brain, it is known as a "focal" seizure. If it spreads to affect the entire brain, it is known as a "generalized" seizure. Focal seizures may be experienced as uncontrolled twitching of a body part without loss of consciousness, whereas generalized seizures are inevitably associated with loss of consciousness and frequently with convulsions throughout the body. Many of the seizures that occur after a stroke start with focal seizure symptoms and then spread through the brain and become generalized, with convulsions and loss of consciousness. Seizures can sometimes present in other ways, such as episodes of unresponsiveness, sometimes with staring, but without shaking or twitching of the body. Some seizures can cause more complicated movements without full loss of consciousness and are known as partial complex seizures. Treatment decisions are based on the type of seizure and the frequency of attacks.

Strokes affecting the outer layers of the brain (cerebral cortex) and those with bleeding into the brain (hemorrhagic strokes) are more likely to cause seizures. In some cases, antiseizure medications (known as "anticonvulsants") will be given as a preventative measure after a stroke that the physician thinks is very likely to result in seizures.

A variety of anticonvulsant medications are available for people who have had seizures after stroke. These include phenytoin (Dilantin), phenobarbital, carbamezapine (Tegretol), valproate (Depakote), and others. All anticonvulsants can cause sedation or interfere with cognitive functioning, though some are more problematic than others. Phenobarbital is notorious for causing drowsiness and exacerbating cognitive problems, and is infrequently used after stroke in the United States for this reason. Dilantin is intermediate in this regard—some tolerate it well, whereas others find it to be sedating. Tegretol and Depakote are generally fairly well tolerated, though some individuals do not react well to them. It is important for family members of patients receiving these drugs to be aware of their potential side effects and report them promptly to the physician. Family members may need to advocate for a trial of an alternative anticonvulsant when they observe cognitive or behavioral side effects that may be subtle.

Seizures can temporarily worsen impairments from a stroke, including "old" impairments that appeared to have resolved. The confusion normally present immediately after a generalized seizure may last longer in a person who has had a prior stroke. Weakness from a stroke that had improved or disappeared commonly returns after a seizure, sometimes for an extended period of time. These neurological symptoms after a seizure may need to be distinguished from a new stroke. Although these temporary neurological impairments typically improve within a few hours, some stroke survivors can experience several days of residual weakness, mild confusion, or other symptoms after a seizure.

Hydrocephalus

The brain is surrounded by a clear protective fluid known as cerebrospinal fluid (CSF). This fluid is produced inside cavities in the middle of the brain known as ventricles. If the flow of the CSF is blocked, fluid can build up inside the brain, causing a condition known as hydrocephalus. Blockage of this flow can be caused by swelling resulting from a stroke, or bleeding into the ventricular system of the brain. When a severe blockage develops suddenly, hydrocephalus can be life-threatening. In less severe or sudden cases, hydrocephalus can lead to more gradual neurological deterioration, with confusion and incontinence common. The treatment of hydrocephalus resulting from stroke depends on the circumstances. In the acute phase, a drain may be placed directly into the ventricle through the skull to relieve the pressure. Longer-term management of hydrocephalus consists of placing a tube from the ventricle to the abdominal cavity, known as a ventriculoperitoneal (VP) shunt. These tubes are tunneled underneath the skin and can usually be felt as they traverse the head, neck, and chest.

VP shunts generally don't require any specific care, though they can become clogged or infected. Family members should be aware of the symptoms of VP shunt malfunction, including headache, visual changes, nausea and vomiting, fever, and confusion or slowed thinking.

Venous Thrombosis

The reduced physical activity that frequently results from a stroke can predispose the patient to developing blood clots in the legs, known as deep venous thrombosis, or DVT. This risk is greatest within the first few weeks after a stroke, and gradually falls over time. The risk is greatest in the weakened leg, though the bed rest that often follows a stroke makes the unaffected leg vulnerable to clots as well. Preventive treatments should be provided starting in the acute care hospital, and continuing through at least several weeks of rehabilitation for people with significant leg weakness after a stroke. Several treatments are available, including the use of pneumatic compression boots, which intermittently squeeze the leg to move the blood back toward the heart, heparin, and heparin-related medications that are injected: Lovenox (enoxaparin), Fragmin (dalteparin), and others. Sometimes the need for DVT prevention dovetails with the need for prevention of another stroke, and the same medication (for example, Coumadin) can serve double duty. DVT can still occur despite preventative treatment. In some cases, symptoms can be mild, and painless swelling may be the only complaint. In other cases, pain, tenderness, and even fever can occur. An ultrasound is usually the diagnostic test of choice for this disorder, though blood tests (d-dimer) are used in some institutions as a screening test. Treatment of a DVT after stroke should usually be continued for at least six months. Elastic stockings may also be helpful to reduce the persistent swelling that can occur after a DVT.

One of the major risks of a DVT is that a clot from the leg will break off and travel to the lungs. This is known as a "pulmonary embolism" and is a serious and potentially life-threatening complication of stroke. Symptoms of pulmonary embolism can be varied, but commonly include chest pain (often worse with a deep breath) and shortness of breath. As with DVT, the best treatment is prevention, and the same treatments are effective as prevention for both DVT and pulmonary embolism. When prevention fails, treatment of pulmonary embolism usually consists of anticoagulation with heparin or related medications (Lovenox) initially, followed by oral treatment with Coumadin for at least six months. In some cases, particularly when anticoagulation poses unacceptable risks (such as shortly after a cerebral hemorrhage), a mechanical filter (a

"Greenfield filter") can be inserted into the main vein carrying blood from the legs to the lungs (known as the inferior vena cava) as a means of physically preventing blood clots from traveling from the legs to the lungs.

Osteoporosis and Fractures

Osteoporosis is the loss of bone (sometimes described as a "thinning" of the bones) that commonly occurs in older people and leads to fractures. Although osteoporosis is often considered a disease of older women, it can affect stroke survivors of both sexes at any age. Bone requires continued active use to maintain its normal strength, and the disuse seen after stroke can lead to osteoporosis in the affected limbs. Unlike osteoporosis seen in older individuals, post-stroke osteoporosis does not usually affect both sides equally, and tends to affect the limbs on the weakened side preferentially. Osteoporosis after stroke can lead to fractures, and the risk of these fractures is heightened by the increased risk of falls in individuals after stroke. The best preventive treatment is regular exercise and use of the affected limbs. Bearing weight on the leg by standing or walking is particularly important.

Medications are commonly used for nonstroke-related osteoporosis but have not been well studied for people with osteoporosis resulting from stroke. The possible use of medication should be discussed with the stroke survivor's physician, particularly in individuals at risk for generalized osteoporosis as well as stroke-related osteoporosis. Adequate intake of calcium and vitamin D is an important preventative measure and should be considered for most individuals.

Edema

The reduced movement commonly present after stroke frequently leads to swelling (edema) of the affected limbs. This is due to the loss of the normal pumping action that occurs with movement and helps remove excess fluid from the limb, as well as the tendency of the stroke survivor to let the affected limb (for example, the hand) "hang down." It is important to be aware that swelling and edema can sometimes be signs of a blood clot in the leg (deep venous thrombosis). Any new swelling should be brought to a physician's attention to assess the possibility of a DVT as the cause.

Post-stroke edema is treated in several ways, often in combination in severe cases. Elevation of the involved extremity is one of the basic interventions to help reduce or even prevent edema. Taking a break in the middle of the day and lying down or elevating the leg or arm can help control edema. At night or when sitting, the arm should be positioned (perhaps on a pillow) so that the elbow is raised somewhat, and the hand is above the elbow.

In cases where elevation is insufficient to control the edema, elastic compression garments can be used. Elastic gloves such as Isotoner gloves can be used for the hand. Elastic stockings, made by Jobst and other companies, can control leg swelling. The white elastic stockings sometimes used to reduce the risk of blood clots ("TED" stockings) in the hospital are of some value but do not provide as much support as the Jobst or similar garments. Elastic bandages, such as Coban wrapping for the hand or Ace bandages for the legs, can also be used, though their use is confined to the rehabilitation hospital because application is so labor-intensive. Massage is another technique that can be quite helpful for hand edema. Generally a physical or occupational therapist will start at the ends of the fingers and work the edema fluid toward the upper arm and chest. Patients and their families can learn this technique as well, and use it at home as another means of controlling edema. Lastly, in cases where hand swelling is accompanied by stiffness, a machine known as a Continuous Passive Motion device, or CPM machine, can be used to move the fingers back and forth repeatedly. Some practitioners have had good results with this device.

These techniques usually provide sufficient control of edema after stroke. In severe cases that do not respond to these treatments, pneumatic compression devices can be used for the arm or leg. These devices are effective but inconvenient and rarely required. Diuretics (medications that cause increased urine production to eliminate fluid, also known as "water pills") are sometimes used in recalcitrant cases of leg edema, but they are not always effective for post-stroke edema and may have side effects.

Skin Problems

Stroke can lead to a variety of skin problems. Early recognition and taking appropriate measures can prevent a small problem from becoming a large one. In the early phase after stroke, the risk of bedsores, also known as "decubitus ulcers," is highest, as mobility is most severely impaired. Frequent turning, keeping the skin dry and clean, avoiding excessive pressure in any single area through appropriate padding (for example, an air mattress overlay), and adequate nutrition are key preventative measures. The risk of decubitus ulcers continues in the home setting and can result from excessive time spent sitting in a wheelchair without relieving the pressure on the buttocks. The preventative measures for home are similar and should include an appropriate wheelchair cushion for individuals spending substantial time seated in a wheelchair, and frequent repositioning.

As a result of reduced movement after stroke, some areas of the skin may not get enough air circulation but too much moisture. This can occur on the inside of the elbow, the hand, or in the groin, among other areas. This excessive moisture can lead to fungal infections, usually manifested as a rash, and sometimes open sores or cracks in the skin. Treatment involves appropriate range-of-motion exercises, and splints in some cases (for the hand). If abnormal increased muscle tone is present (spasticity), treatment of the underlying spasticity may be beneficial in protecting the skin. Antifungal creams such as clotrimazole (Lotrimin) may be needed to treat these rashes in conjunction with providing a clean, dry environment.

Pneumonia

Pneumonia often complicates stroke care in the hospital, but it tends to be less common as recovery from the stroke progresses. A major factor in the development of pneumonia is swallowing difficulty (dysphagia), and many cases of post-stroke pneumonia result from "aspiration," in which food or oral secretions are inhaled into the lung and cause an infection. Early recognition of swallowing difficulties and avoiding feeding until swallowing has recovered sufficiently are important preventative measures, though they are not 100 percent protective. Treatment for pneumonia after stroke includes antibiotics, chest physical therapy in some cases, and oxygen if needed.

Sleep Disturbance

Sleep is often disrupted early after a stroke—particularly while the patient is still hospitalized. Disruptions of the normal sleep-wake cycle are common in individuals with cognitive impairments after a stroke, and in severe cases they can result in reversal of the perception of day and night. People whose sleep-wake cycle is altered may sleep much of the day and be awake much of the night—a pattern not very conducive to rehabilitation efforts. These sleep-wake cycle disturbances exacerbate any existing cognitive impairments and worsen symptoms of confusion.

Behavioral approaches to managing sleep-wake cycle disturbances are the best choice. These include providing adequate stimulation during the daytime (including keeping the patient out of bed as much as possible), avoiding daytime naps, and establishing a quiet, undistracted environment for sleep at night (often difficult to achieve in a hospital setting). In cases where behavioral approaches are not sufficient to reestablish a normal sleep pattern, medications are often used. There are two basic kinds of medications, and they can be used individually or in combination: medications to help with sleep at night and stimulant medications to increase alertness during the day. Sleep medications include diazepam (Valium) and its many related medications, including temazepam (Restoril), oxazepam (Serax), alprazolam (Xanax), and others; zolpidem (Ambien), zaleplon (Sonata); and antidepressant medications with sedating effects, such as trazadone (Desyrel), nefazadone (Serzone), and others. In general, sleeping medications should be used sparingly, since the more frequently they are used, the less effective they become. Moreover, use of these medications can result in persistent sedation in the morning. Longer-acting medications such as Valium should generally be avoided for this reason.

Stimulant medications include methylphenidate (Ritalin), dextroamphetamine (Dexedrine), modafinil (Provigil), and others. These medications may have other associated benefits in some stroke survivors, such as improving attention or overall alertness. If given too late in the day these medications can cause insomnia. In higher doses many of these medications can also suppress appetite—an undesirable side effect in a stroke survivor.

Sleep-wake cycle disturbances typically resolve as a new routine is established; they are rarely a long-term problem after stroke. In the long run, behavioral approaches are generally the most effective.

Sleep Apnea

Another common sleep disturbance after stroke is sleep apnea. Apnea is the medical term for failure to breathe, and individuals with sleep apnea have episodes during sleep when breathing stops. The most common form of sleep apnea is obstructive sleep apnea, which can occur in people who have never had a stroke but is even more common after stroke. Obstructive sleep apnea is caused by the tissues in the back of the throat blocking the breathing passageway during sleep. This condition is most common in overweight individuals with short necks, and is more common in men than in women. Many individuals with this type of apnea have a history of severe snoring, which can serve as another clue in diagnosing this condition.

When people with obstructive sleep apnea stop breathing, they automatically partially wake up due to the body's protective systems that guard against suffocating while asleep. Often the person with apnea does not realize that he's having these episodes, but a spouse or roommate can frequently identify these symptoms. Because the individual is waking up so often, he never achieves deep enough sleep to become rested, and often has difficulty staying awake during the day. Treatment usually involves a special mask and device known as a "CPAP" machine to help "push" air in during the night and keep the airways open.

Occasionally, two other forms of breathing disturbance can occur after stroke: central sleep apnea and Cheyne-Stokes respiration. Central sleep apnea is a condition in which the brain does not send the signals to breathe as often as it should during sleep. This can result in decreased oxygen levels in the blood during sleep and drowsiness during the day, similar to obstructive sleep apnea. In Cheyne-Stokes respiration, the signals from the brain to breathe develop a cyclical pattern, with episodes of apnea followed by episodes of rapid breathing. Oxygen levels fall during the episodes of apnea. Treatment with theophylline is sometimes used for these central sleep disturbances, though its efficacy is uncertain. Nocturnal oxygen therapy may also be useful.

Fatigue

Fatigue is a very common symptom after stroke, though little is known about the exact cause. For some individuals, sleep problems are a contributing factor (see above), but for many, there is no obvious cause other than the stroke itself. Fatigue tends to be most severe early after a stroke and gradually improve over time. Some individuals find that their energy level never quite gets back to normal, however, even many years after a stroke. Severe fatigue can also make neurological symptoms more pronounced. For example, a person with dysarthria after a stroke may find that her speech becomes more slurred late in the day when she is fatigued.

Planning for rest periods during the day, including short naps if needed, is generally the best approach for managing fatigue. Occasionally, stimulant medications such as Ritalin (methylphenidate) seem to benefit severely affected individuals.

6

Recovery and Rehabilitation

Louise and Mary are both women in their mid-seventies who find themselves hospital roommates after experiencing strokes within a few hours of
each other. Louise suddenly developed right-hand weakness and slurred
speech. Her physician tells her that she has had a "small" stroke affecting
mostly the motor functions to her right hand and speech articulation.
Mary, by contrast, has severe weakness of her entire left side. She is told by
her physician that she has had a large stroke affecting the right hemisphere
of the brain.

Over the next few days, Louise finds that her hand is gradually recovering and her speech is steadily improving. Mary, however, finds little change over the same time period. Louise is discharged directly
home from the hospital and ultimately has a near complete recovery.
Mary, on the other hand, is transferred to a rehabilitation hospital. She
never regains useful movement in her arm and only limited movement
in her leg.

The cases of Louise and Mary raise a number of important questions:
Can the brain heal itself? How much recovery will a person experience
after a stroke? What can someone do to maximize the amount of recovery?

Despite the importance of these questions, the answers are still only
partially known. Substantial recovery frequently occurs after stroke but is
often incomplete. Although physicians have worked to develop tools to
help them predict recovery, it is still difficult to foresee how much someone will recover. What we do know is that recovery is not a "passive" pro-

cess but one that, if it is to be successful, requires the active participation of the patient and, ideally, his loved ones as well.

The terms "rehabilitation" and "recovery" are often used together. Although the two processes are closely connected, there are important distinctions between them. "Recovery" is best defined as the actual return of neurological function after stroke. Regaining normal use of a weak arm after stroke is an example of recovery. Everyone (patients, family, and healthcare providers) would like to see as much recovery occur as possible, and hence a return to the state of health the stroke survivor enjoyed before her illness. Recovery is often incomplete, however, despite our efforts to stimulate this process. Future research on stimulating recovery should continue to identify new and more effective approaches to restoring neurological function.

Since recovery is often incomplete, stroke survivors need to learn skills to manage in spite of altered neurological function. These skills are often termed "compensation." Compensation takes a variety of forms, some more obvious than others. For someone who has lost the use of an arm, a compensatory strategy might include learning how to button his clothing using one-handed techniques. Another example of compensation would be learning exercises to strengthen the unaffected leg for someone who sustains leg weakness after a stroke. This increased strength may help walking ability, despite the fact that the original weakness has not changed.

"Rehabilitation" encompasses both recovery and compensation. Rehabilitation is the process of helping someone who has had a stroke regain her ability to function in daily life and society. This includes taking advantage of spontaneous recovery, stimulating further recovery to the extent possible, and teaching compensatory strategies to fill in the gaps. Rehabilitation is a very important part of the process of resuming a satisfying and full life after a stroke.

Neurological Recovery

Neurological recovery usually begins within the first few days after a stroke and may be quite rapid in some cases. Recovery appears to occur through a number of mechanisms. In some cases, there is substantial swelling (edema) of the brain surrounding the area of the stroke, and it gradually returns to normal over a period of days to weeks. This edema is particularly prominent in cerebral hemorrhages. Often an area around the perimeter of the stroke has experienced a partial loss of blood flow. Once blood flow is restored, portions of this area, known as the ischemic penumbra, may recover from the injury and regain normal functioning.

The brain has many interconnections between different functional areas. The sudden loss of activity and "input" from an area of the brain affected by stroke can cause loss of function in an area physically remote from the damage site. This phenomenon is known as diaschisis. It is somewhat analogous to an automobile factory in which shutting down the section that fabricates the transmissions may lead to temporarily shutting down the areas where the drive train is assembled. Diaschisis often improves as the remote areas of the brain learn to compensate for the lost activity and input that formerly came from the area damaged by the stroke.

Unfortunately, the brain cannot regenerate or "grow back" areas that have been lost as a result of stroke. Nonetheless, the brain has mechanisms for restructuring itself to recover somewhat from the aftereffects of a stroke. Older views of the brain as a static organ incapable of change once a person reaches adulthood have been turned upside down in recent years. The brain's ability to adapt is known as "plasticity." We know that the brain undergoes adaptive changes after a stroke even without specific treatments. Increasingly, however, we are learning that this process can be enhanced by specific activities, with the result of improved function.

In plasticity, new connections form between brain cells. Through this process of "rewiring," areas that were not damaged by the stroke take over the responsibilities of the areas that have been lost. This is most marked in small strokes, where this ability may be sufficient, over time, to completely overcome the effects of the stroke. In larger strokes, however, the adjacent areas of the brain may also be severely affected by the stroke. More distant areas may lack the connections needed to assume the lost functions, and may already be specialized in other key brain functions. In some cases, a different mechanism is used by the brain to adapt to the damage it has sustained. In these cases, some of the lost functions are taken over by the "matching" or equivalent area on the opposite side of the brain from the stroke. While the general principle is that the right side of the brain controls the left side of the body and vice versa, the reality is a bit more complex. Even in people without any history of stroke or other neurological disorder, there are connections between each side of the brain and the same side of the body, though fewer than those between each side of the brain and the opposite side of the body. It seems that these "same-side" connections may be able to take over some of the functions of the damaged side of the brain. Thus after a stroke affecting the left side of the brain, the right side may assume some of the control of movement of the right side of the body.

The relative importance of each of these mechanisms of recovery varies on the basis of the nature of the stroke and perhaps other, as yet unknown, factors.

How long after a stroke can recovery take place? Surprisingly, we don't know the answer to this question. In the past, it was assumed that the possibility of neurological recovery ended within a few months after stroke. More recently, however, scientists are questioning this assumption. Research showing improvements with exercise training even years after a stroke has opened the possibility that some recovery may be long-lasting. Despite this encouraging news, the fact remains that most recovery takes place within the first few months after a stroke.

Neurogenesis

In an important new discovery, scientists have recently found that the human brain can produce new brain cells (neurons). We don't yet know the extent to which this is possible, but it is clear that at least some areas of the brain are capable of producing new brain cells (neurogenesis) throughout adulthood and even into old age. At the same time, this ability appears to be limited and does not include the regrowth of damaged brain tissue. Some scientists have proposed stimulating this capability in some fashion to improve recovery after stroke. Although this is not yet feasible, it is an extremely important and exciting area of research.

Growth Factors

Other techniques to help the brain recover after stroke have been proposed and studied to varying degrees. One approach is to use chemicals that stimulate the cells within the brain to form more connections to other brain cells. The idea behind this treatment strategy is that forming more connections after a stroke may allow the brain to "rewire" itself more effectively to recover lost functions. These chemicals, known as "growth factors," are normally produced in the brain in small quantities. By identifying them and producing larger amounts in the laboratory, neuroscientists hope to discover growth factors helpful in stimulating recovery after stroke.

Stem Cells

Stem cells are cells within the body that retain the ability to produce a variety of different specialized cell types needed by the body. Stem cells have received considerable attention in the media in recent months owing to controversy over the use of fetal tissue for research purposes. The ethical debate concerns stem cells that are obtained from aborted fetuses or from embryos produced in the laboratory using in vitro fertilization techniques. But these are not the only sources of stem cells; research has increasingly identified stem cells in adults as well. It is conceivable that by placing a person's own stem cells in the area of the brain damaged by stroke, we might further enhance recovery. Despite the obvious appeal of this approach, it has not yet been shown to be workable or effective. A variety of theoretical and technical problems must be solved before this treatment becomes standard after stroke.

Medications

Medications have also been used to improve brain recovery after stroke. The most promising of these are stimulant medications known as amphetamines and related compounds. Dexedrine (dextroamphetamine) has been shown in some preliminary studies to stimulate recovery of motor abilities when combined with physical therapy. Other studies have looked at similar medications, such as Ritalin (methylphenidate). Currently these medications are used after stroke for other purposes—most typically for problems focusing and maintaining attention (see Chapter 13). Larger, more definitive research studies are under way to determine if these medications are truly helpful in promoting recovery after stroke.

Exercise for Recovery

Recovery of movement after stroke is clearly a key goal for many stroke survivors and their families. Animal studies have provided important insights into the influence of activity on the recovery process for weakness after stroke. In one experiment, strokes were induced in animals, who were then placed in one of two groups. In one group, the animals had their weak forelimbs placed in a restrictive splint so they couldn't use the limbs during the first few weeks after their stroke. In the other group, the animals were allowed to move about freely and use the limbs as much as they were able. The animals that weren't allowed to use their limbs did not recover as much movement as the animals that had free use of their weak limbs. This study demonstrated that activity is important to recovering function after a stroke.

A similar experiment looked at stroke in rats. Half of the rats were allowed to move around normally in their cages, whereas the other half were given a special cage with increased activities available (for example, a wheel and mazes to run in). The enriched environment provided to these rats can be thought of as a sort of "rat rehabilitation" program. These animals recovered more movement than those that did not have access to extra activities.

On the basis of these and other animal studies, most physicians and scientists agree that exercise and activity enhance recovery. Research examining the use of exercise to promote stroke recovery in humans is discussed in Chapter 11.

The Process of Rehabilitation

For many stroke survivors, rehabilitation is a long and multistaged process. Navigating this complex and often unfamiliar part of the healthcare system is challenging and requires some understanding of the components of rehabilitation and the settings in which they are provided.

In an ideal world, all decisions regarding medical care would be based solely on the needs of the patient, and all stroke survivors would receive the best possible rehabilitation care. In reality, many factors affect the provision of rehabilitation care after stroke, including insurance coverage, controversies regarding the efficacy of various interventions, geographic and cultural considerations, physician preference, patient and family preference, and many others. While there is no clear definition of what constitutes the ideal rehabilitation program, some general guidelines are provided here that should aid stroke survivors and their families in their decision-making. Family advocacy can play a critical role in obtaining the optimal rehabilitation program for a stroke survivor, as will be further described below.

Rehabilitation in the Acute Care Hospital

Rehabilitation activities should begin as soon as possible after a stroke. At first, these may be focused on assessment and prevention of complications rather than on restoration of function. For example, a speech therapist may be called upon to assess swallowing function and the safety of resuming eating. If there is ankle weakness, a physical therapist may provide a splint to keep the ankle in a favorable position. If the patient has experienced mild loss of balance after a stroke, a physical therapist may practice walking with him so he can return directly home from the hospital.

Because of the short duration of most acute care hospitalizations after stroke, rehabilitation efforts in this phase of care are usually limited in scope and duration. The next phase of rehabilitation is determined during the acute care hospitalization, however, so that's the time for the patient and family members to ensure that optimal rehabilitation care is arranged. Unfortunately, loved ones often have little time to investigate rehabilitation options owing to the pressure to move stroke patients out of the acute care hospital as soon as they are medically stabilized. Family members should begin investigating rehabilitation options in their area as soon as possible after the patient is admitted to the hospital, and engage both the physician and the case manager assigned by the hospital in a discussion of options after discharge. Physical, occupational, and speech therapists, as well as nurses on the stroke/neurology floor, may also be a helpful source of information regarding rehabilitation facilities in the area. Planning post-hospitalization rehabilitation as early in the hospital stay as possible will help avoid a hasty choice of the first available facility rather than selection of the best one available.

Inpatient (Hospital-Level) Rehabilitation

A freestanding rehabilitation hospital or a rehabilitation hospital unit located within an acute care hospital generally provides the most comprehensive and intensive rehabilitation services post-stroke. These programs are designed to provide at least three hours of rehabilitation therapies each day, in addition to making available nurses and physicians specializing in stroke rehabilitation. Physicians are usually trained in physical medicine and rehabilitation (a medical specialty devoted to rehabilitation), neurology, or occasionally other rehabilitation-related specialties. They are typically highly involved in the rehabilitation process, visiting patients at least three to five times per week. The physical, occupational, and speech therapists on these units are usually employed full-time at the rehabilitation hospital/unit, and they all meet regularly with nurses and the physician to review each patient's progress and rehabilitation program.

The average stay at inpatient rehabilitation units is about three weeks for stroke survivors, though there is significant variability from facility to facility and from patient to patient. Since this level of care is relatively expensive, some insurance companies provide limited benefits or may not provide coverage at all. This type of care remains the "gold standard" for moderate to severe strokes, however, and family members may need to advocate for this level of care when it is needed.

A variant of this type of care is the "long-term acute care" or "LTAC" hospital or hospital unit. These hospital-level programs typically are capable of providing a high degree of medical management. There is considerable variation among these hospitals, with some providing the same scope of rehabilitation services as a rehabilitation hospital, and others more focused on specialized medical care, such as treatment of patients requiring mechanical ventilators.

Obtaining reliable and meaningful information to help guide the selection of a hospital-level rehabilitation program can be challenging.

Some programs (particularly freestanding rehabilitation hospitals) may have web sites that provide some information about the program. Families should inquire about the staffing of the program, including professional background of physicians and whether or not they are devoted to the program full-time. Most high-quality programs are accredited as rehabilitation programs through a voluntary organization known as CARF (the Committee on Accreditation of Rehabilitation Facilities). Most high-quality programs collect data on their outcomes, which may be available on request. Comparing data from different facilities can be difficult, however, because patient populations sometimes vary. Often decisions regarding rehabilitation programs are based on local reputation—this is not a perfect measure of a good program, but often it is the best available.

Skilled Nursing Facilities

Skilled nursing facilities, sometimes known as SNFs, provide a highly variable level of rehabilitation services. Some skilled nursing facilities have relatively robust and well-organized short-term rehabilitation programs, whereas others may provide limited rehabilitation therapy services with little coordinated management of the rehabilitation program. Physician involvement is usually substantially less than in a rehabilitation hospital, and physician care may not be provided by a physician specializing in stroke rehabilitation.

In addition to short-term rehabilitative care, skilled nursing facilities usually (though not always) provide long-term residential care for individuals who are unable to return to the community. In some cases the short-term rehabilitation-oriented program and long-term care program are intermingled; in others they are housed on separate units.

Skilled nursing facilities may be appropriate choices for individuals with relatively mild strokes who are anticipating a short stay and have fairly modest rehabilitation needs, or for individuals who are so severely affected that they are not expected to benefit much from rehabilitation. For patients with intermediate levels of impairment from stroke, I believe rehabilitation hospitals generally offer a more comprehensive approach. Some skilled nursing facilities provide excellent rehabilitative care, however, and are deserving of consideration as an alternative.

Skilled nursing facilities are also appropriate in some cases as an intermediate step between a rehabilitation hospital stay and return home. A short stay in an SNF may allow further time for recovery and rehabilitation in some individuals and facilitate return to the community. In other cases, long-term nursing home care may be required owing to the severity of the stroke and the inability of a family to provide the extensive supportive care needed at home.

Before selecting a skilled nursing facility for short-term rehabilitative care, family members should investigate how much therapy is provided, how the rehabilitation process is managed, and whether physicians with expertise in stroke rehabilitation are available to help manage the rehabilitation process. These resources may be particularly important if a person is having difficulty achieving her rehabilitation potential. A visit to the skilled nursing facility may be helpful in assessing the stroke rehabilitation care provided there.

In cases where long-term nursing home care is required, families should be sure to visit the specific unit where their family member is likely to reside. Cleanliness, staffing levels, staff attitudes, medical coverage, amenities for residents, and physical surroundings are all important factors to assess. The U.S. government now provides detailed information regarding nursing home performance and outcomes on a publicly available web site: http://www.medicare.gov/nhcompare/home.asp. This site provides a wealth of information about past performance. A major caveat when using this data is that the nursing home industry is very unstable, with frequent changes in management. It is important to inquire about recent changes in management and staffing since the most recent data were posted.

Transitional Care Units

Transitional care units (sometimes abbreviated TCUs) are skilled nursing facilities located within an acute care hospital. These units are generally oriented toward short stays only and do not have a long-term residential component. Because they are located in a hospital setting, these units generally have frequent physician availability and structured rehabilitation programs. They often function as intermediate levels of rehabilitation, with less intensity than a rehabilitation hospital but more intensive rehabilitation services than a skilled nursing facility located in the community. As a result of changes in the reimbursement system, TCUs are less widely available now than in the past.

Home Care

Some stroke survivors are fortunate enough to be able to return directly home. Others, as discussed above, may require another stop (for example, a rehabilitation hospital) before returning home. Many stroke survivors from both of these groups, however, will require home care services to help them adjust to living back at home. Home care agencies (also known as visiting nurse agencies) are organizations devoted to providing this type of care. Many are affiliated with hospitals or hospital systems, whereas others are independent organizations. The keystone of home care is the visiting nurse. Even for individuals with minimal nursing needs, the nurse serves an important role in coordinating care at home and trouble-shooting any problems. The nurse can provide education and assistance with a variety of tasks that may seem daunting to stroke survivors and their families after return home. Educating patients and family members on the administration of injectable medications (such as insulin), instructing them how to use tube feedings for individuals with swallowing difficulties, and monitoring the use and effects of medications such as Coumadin (warfarin) are just some of the things visiting nurses do.

One of the peculiarities of home care is the requirement by Medicare (and often other health insurers as well) that someone be "homebound" in order to receive these services. This generally means that all rehabilitation therapy and nursing services must be provided either at home *or* in the outpatient setting. "Mixing and matching" outpatient and home care services is generally not allowed by insurers. The logic appears to be that if you are able to leave the home for some services, you are no longer homebound, and so no longer qualify for home care services. This can cause difficulties for individuals who would prefer outpatient rehabilitative services but have nursing needs that can only be managed at home. Some private insurance companies have more flexible rules and may allow mixing home and outpatient services.

Home care services may also include assistance with daily tasks from a home health aide. Assistance with bathing, for example, may be provided. These services are usually for a short period of time each day. Aides are not intended to provide extended supervision and care during the day.

The home care services supplied by Medicare and other insurers do not provide adequate assistance to people unable to care for themselves. These services are also typically only provided for a relatively short period of time to assist in the transition home. Someone who has been severely disabled after a stroke needs additional services so family members can return to work or other responsibilities.

Some families are fortunate enough to be able to afford privately hired personal-care attendants for more extensive assistance at home. Personal-care attendants (PCAs) can be hired through an agency or directly from the community. Agency staff are usually available on relatively short notice but tend to be more expensive than privately hired PCAs. Hiring one or more PCAs privately reduces the cost but provides less backup for absences and requires a greater effort to set up. PCAs are not licensed personnel and may have little medical training or experience. Agencies typically limit the scope of duties for PCAs working within their organization, whereas privately hired PCAs may be more flexible in assisting with certain medically oriented tasks (such as helping with a feeding tube or urinary catheter). Strategies for identifying PCA candidates outside an agency include using help wanted ads in local newspapers, networking through church groups, or asking friends or work contacts if they know of anyone. When hiring a PCA, it is usually helpful to include an orientation period during which the person can receive instruction and education in the specific needs of the patient.

In cases where a stroke survivor in need of these services lives far away from her family, a privately hired care manager may be helpful, though this adds another layer of expense. Care managers coordinate the care programs for a disabled person living alone, including finding personal-care attendants, making arrangements in cases where an attendant is unexpectedly unavailable due to illness, and organizing medical care and transportation. These services are relatively new and vary in quality and cost. There is currently no license required for this position. The National Association of Professional Geriatric Care Managers (www.caremanager.org) can help you find a local care manager. The Eldercare Locator (www.eldercare.gov) managed by the U.S. Administration on Aging also provides local links for consumers seeking to identify services in their area.

Outpatient Services

Outpatient rehabilitation services (sometimes termed "ambulatory services") are generally appropriate for people who are medically stable, still require active rehabilitation, and are able to travel from home to an outpatient facility. Most individuals requiring these services will travel to a hospital-based outpatient facility or a freestanding rehabilitation center. Some people require a more structured day program for their outpatient rehabilitation. This may include stroke survivors who have cognitive impairments and are not able to direct their own care safely, and whose families are not available throughout the day to provide supervision and care. Day programs encompass a comprehensive set of rehabilitation services, though they may rely more heavily on group-therapy treatments than would a conventional individualized outpatient rehabilitation program. Some institutions have "day hospital" programs that seek to replicate the intensity of inpatient rehabilitation care for individuals who are stable enough medically to stay in the community with their families.

Adult Day Care

Adult day care programs provide supervision and socialization for individuals who are living in the community and have completed their formal rehabilitation. These programs may be helpful for stroke survivors who were previously in a rehabilitation day program or for relatively independent older people who are seeking social support in a community setting.

Who Works in an Inpatient Program?

Rehabilitation programs are usually highly structured and involve multiple medical disciplines. Each program is staffed a bit differently. Rehabilitation is a team effort, with therapists, physicians, nurses, patient, and family all playing key roles. The more effectively the team works together, the more efficiently the rehabilitation goals will be achieved. What follows is a general guide to in-house rehabilitation professionals.

Physicians

The role of the physician is to manage medical issues that arise during the course of rehabilitation, as well as to lead the rehabilitation team. The physician reviews the medical plan for preventing another stroke and ensures that an appropriate evaluation for the cause of the stroke has been completed. Medical conditions, including hypertension, diabetes, and any complications of stroke are managed by the physician. Any physician consultations, such as a cardiology evaluation, are ordered by the physician, as well as any diagnostic tests needed, such as an x-ray swallowing study. Several different kinds of specialists may serve as attending physicians on a rehabilitation unit, and in some cases, a shared management model is in use, whereby two physicians of different specialties co-manage the medical care (for example, an internist and a physiatrist). Medical specialties most commonly involved in stroke rehabilitation include physical medicine and rehabilitation (physiatry), neurology, and internal medicine.

PHYSIATRISTS

Physiatrists are physicians specializing in the medical care and rehabilitation of individuals with disabling conditions such as stroke. Physicians in this specialty generally complete a four-year training program, which includes one year of general medical training (often in internal medicine), and three years of training in physical medicine and rehabilitation. Training in this specialty includes experience in managing a broad range of disabling conditions, working with a rehabilitation team, using exercise as a treatment, prescribing braces and splints, and managing spasticity.

Physiatrists provide care for stroke survivors beyond the hospital stay. They can help address the long-term complications and rehabilitative needs that can arise long after the patient has returned home from the hospital.

NEUROLOGISTS

Neurologists are physicians specializing in the diagnosis and treatment of disorders of the nervous system. Neurologists receive specific training in the diagnosis and treatment of acute stroke and in the prevention of recurrent stroke. Some neurologists obtain additional training specifically in neurorehabilitation during a fellowship after their residency training has been completed.

INTERNISTS

Internists are physicians specializing in the diagnosis and treatment of adults with a broad range of medical problems affecting the organ systems of the body. Many internists also undergo subspecialty training in areas such as geriatrics, cardiology, and pulmonary medicine, among others.

RESIDENTS AND OTHER MEDICAL TRAINEES

Some rehabilitation programs are training sites for physicians. These may include medical students, residents, and fellows. Medical students are at an early point in their training and are usually closely supervised. Residents have completed medical school and are obtaining training in their chosen specialty (for example, physical medicine and rehabilitation). Fellows have completed their training in a medical specialty (say, neurology) and have chosen to obtain further subspecialty training. In general, the level of autonomy provided to these trainees increases with the level of their training. Advantages of receiving care in a facility with a training program include the ability of these programs to attract excellent physicians, and a tendency to be on the forefront of advances in the field of rehabilitation.

Physician Assistants

Physician assistants (PAs) work with physicians and may be present on the rehabilitation unit when the physician is unavailable. Physician assistants generally function as a physician "extender." They prescribe medications, order diagnostic tests, and obtain consultations from physicians in other specialties as appropriate.

Nurses

Nurses play a key role in the rehabilitation process. In fact, individuals undergoing rehabilitation spend more time with nursing staff than with any other member of the rehabilitation team. Nurses administer medications, assess patient medical status, and determine the significance of any change in condition. Nurses help patients reestablish control over their bowels and bladders, work on their mobility and activities of daily living, and ensure adequate nutrition. Nurses play a key role in educating patients and their families about the practical aspects of living with the aftereffects of a stroke. Some nurses receive special certification in rehabilitation nursing and devote themselves to this specialty.

NURSING AIDES (NAs) AND CERTIFIED NURSING ASSISTANTS (CNAs)

Nursing aides and nursing assistants are highly involved in the daily care of stroke survivors while they are in the hospital or rehabilitation facility. They work with the nursing staff to provide help with toileting, feeding, dressing, and other daily tasks.

Nurse Practitioners

Nurse practitioners are nurses who have received advanced training and are qualified to provide medical care under the supervision of a collaborating physician. Nurse practitioners may order medications and laboratory tests. They function with considerable autonomy in providing medical care.

Physical Therapists

Physical Therapists (PTs) are trained in providing exercise and related treatments to enhance mobility and functional independence. Physical therapists perform much of the "hands-on" work associated with learning how to get out of bed, manage a wheelchair if appropriate, and/or return to walking as feasible. PTs have extensive training in the mechanics and physiology of movement, as well as expertise in the use of braces, wheelchairs, and ambulatory aides. Physical therapists play a major role in the restoration of independence after a stroke.

PHYSICAL THERAPY ASSISTANTS (PTAs) AND AIDES

Physical therapy assistants provide care similar to that provided by physical therapists, though there are limits to how much they can do owing to their more limited training. PTAs generally work under the direction of a

physical therapist, though they may function with considerable autonomy. Physical therapy aides provide exercise therapy under the direction
of a physical therapist.

Occupational Therapists

Occupational therapists (OTs) provide treatment to enhance a patient's
ability to perform activities of daily living. These activities include bathing, dressing, using the toilet, feeding, and cooking. Because the hand
is used so extensively in these activities, occupational therapists devote
more time to the arm and hand than do other therapists. Occupational
therapy addresses the cognitive effects of stroke, particularly as they relate to daily activities. Physical mobility also plays a key role in the tasks
of daily life, so OTs work on mobility issues as well. They coordinate their
activities closely with the rest of the rehabilitation team to maximize the
independence of the person receiving stroke rehabilitation.

OCCUPATIONAL THERAPY ASSISTANTS (COTAs, OR CERTIFIED OCCUPATIONAL THERAPY ASSISTANTS) AND AIDES

Occupational therapy assistants provide many of the same treatments
as occupational therapists, though with a somewhat narrower range of
practice. COTAs generally work under the direction of an occupational
therapist. Occupational therapy aides provide more limited occupational
therapy treatments under the direction of an occupational therapist.

Speech Language Pathologists

Speech and language pathologists (also known as SLPs or speech therapists) provide therapy for speech and communication disorders, cognitive disorders, and swallowing difficulties. SLPs work with individuals
with aphasia to reestablish effective communication and improve the
quality of speech. They also work with people who have dysarthria to improve the intelligibility of speech, and with people who have language
disorders to help them improve reading and writing skills. SLPs perform
detailed evaluations of swallowing on the basis of examination and testing the ability to swallow foods of varying consistencies. In individuals
with swallowing difficulties, they provide exercises to improve swallow-

ing and teach strategies to make swallowing safer. For stroke survivors with cognitive issues (for example, attention or memory problems), SLPs work to determine the extent of the impairments and then develop corrective and compensatory strategies.

SPEECH TECHNICIANS

Speech technicians work under the direction of an SLP and provide specific treatments under their supervision.

Recreational Therapists

Recreational therapists work with stroke survivors to enhance their quality of life and functional independence through participation in recreational activities. These include gardening, fishing, playing cards, and sports, to name a few. Although some activities are simply intended to make the hospital stay less onerous (for example, showing a movie on the rehabilitation unit), most activities also have the therapeutic goal of restoring abilities affected by the stroke. Recreational therapists are an important resource for patients returning to the community. They can help stroke survivors by facilitating their participation in community-based recreational activities.

Rehabilitation Aides

Rehabilitation aides provide a broad range of assistance to individuals undergoing stroke rehabilitation. Their duties often overlap with those of physical and occupational therapy aides as well as nursing assistants.

Respiratory Therapists

Respiratory therapists assist stroke patients who have breathing issues, such as those with a tracheostomy tube, sleep apnea, or asthma.

Nutritionists

Nutritionists, also known as registered dieticians, provide supervision of appropriate diets in the hospital or other rehabilitation facility, and also play an important role in educating patients and families about special diets. They are an important resource for individuals with dysphagia and special diets, as well as those with other dietary restrictions (such as limited Vitamin K consumption for those receiving Coumadin).

Case Managers

Case managers assist in the coordination and management of the rehabilitation program. Case managers are often nurses by training, though they may be social workers or members of other disciplines as well. Case managers may be employed by a hospital, insurance company, or physician practice, or they may be hired by a patient or patient's family. Their role varies widely depending on their employer. A hospital case manager will often serve as a liaison to the patient's family, providing information about the progress and anticipated goals of rehabilitation. She may also communicate with the insurance company, providing information regarding the expected duration of rehabilitation, and sometimes justifying a continued stay on the rehabilitation unit. An insurance company case manager may monitor utilization of rehabilitation services, as well as provide information to the care team regarding the availability of specific insurance benefits and resources. Occasionally, families will hire their own case managers to help coordinate care in the home setting.

Social Workers

Social workers (MSWs and LCSWs) help patients and their families cope with the aftermath of stroke. Social workers provide counseling services, identify resources in the community, and may facilitate peer support groups for stroke survivors. In some institutions, they may serve as case managers as well (see above).

Neuropsychologists

Neuropsychologists are experts in the cognitive and language aspects of brain functioning. They are often called upon to provide detailed assessments after a stroke. In some rehabilitation programs, they play a role in directing therapy and may also provide direct therapy themselves to cognitively impaired individuals.

Psychologists

Psychologists are experts in the emotional and psychological issues that stroke survivors and their families face. They provide diagnostic and counseling services. Psychologists are commonly involved in cases of post-stroke adjustment difficulties or mild depression. In more severe cases of depression, psychiatrists (physicians specializing in emotional and psychiatric disorders) may become involved to prescribe medications to treat these disorders.

Orthotists

Orthotists are professionals who fit and fabricate braces. A patient who requires a brace after a stroke will generally have a prescription provided by her physician, at which point she will be evaluated by an orthotist. After taking measurements or molds (usually fiberglass casts) of the leg, the orthotist will either fabricate a custom-made brace or provide an "off-the-shelf" prefabricated brace as appropriate. The orthotist will then ensure that the brace fits and functions well, and provide any needed adjustments, maintenance, or repairs in the future. Some rehabilitation facilities employ orthotists directly, whereas many others work with outside vendors to provide their services. The orthotist may see patients in his own office or in a rehabilitation facility clinic, often in a multidisciplinary program with a physician and/or a physical therapist participating.

Pedorthotists

Pedorthotists are trained in the provision of orthopedic and other medically necessary shoes and foot orthotics.

Vocational Counselors

Vocational counselors are trained in evaluating an individual's ability to work and providing counseling and guidance to those seeking to return to the workforce. Vocational counselors can serve as a liaison to a current employer, as well as help define realistic goals for return to work. In cases where return to a prior position is not realistic, vocational counselors can help set up retraining opportunities to allow return to more suitable employment.

Rehabilitation and Recovery Timetable

One of the first questions stroke survivors and their families ask is, "How long will it take for me/my loved one to get better?" The answer to this question depends on a number of factors and varies from person to person.

Generally speaking, neurological recovery begins almost immediately after a stroke. The most rapid recovery usually takes place in the first few weeks and months after a stroke, with the largest amount of recovery occurring within the first three to six months. The second six months after a stroke are usually a time of slower improvement, but recovery can continue in many cases for up to one year.

Certain aspects of recovery seem to proceed on a different timetable. The recovery from aphasia or from cognitive effects of a stroke may be slower and more prolonged than recovery from other impairments. I have cared for a number of patients who have had meaningful improvements in these areas in the second year after a stroke.

Individuals who have a cerebral hemorrhage seem to have a somewhat slower and more prolonged recovery process than those with an infarct. Research in this area is limited, but it seems that the overall outcomes are fairly similar between people who have had cerebral hemorrhages and those with infarcts.

Individual experiences vary widely, of course. Equally important, our understanding of the ability to modify recovery with exercise or other treatments is still in its infancy. It seems clear already, however, that these new treatments may extend the period of recovery beyond the estimates given here.

Recovery and rehabilitation cannot be rushed. The brain, like all human organs, requires time to heal itself. While rehabilitation efforts need to be sufficiently intensive to stimulate the brain's recovery, there is likely a point of diminishing returns, when further increases in therapy time do not provide further benefit. Moreover, if therapy is too intensive, fatigue or exhaustion may reduce a person's ability to focus attention and energy on rehabilitation efforts. "Tincture of time," that is, giving the body a chance to heal itself, is a time-honored medical prescription for many ailments. Stroke rehabilitation is no exception.

Rehabilitation and recovery operate on distinct timetables, though the two processes overlap. Initial rehabilitation efforts often begin in the acute hospital, where length of stay after a stroke may only be a few days in uncomplicated cases. Rehabilitation hospital stays have been steadily shrinking and now average approximately three weeks. There is considerable variation around this duration, however; some mildly affected individuals may stay one week in a rehabilitation hospital whereas those with complicated cases may stay six or eight weeks. Length of stay in skilled nursing facilities is often governed in large part by insurance benefits and usually varies from two weeks to three months for short-term rehabilitative care (in contrast, long-term nursing home stays can be indefinite).

The duration of home-based services has been shrinking as a result of pressure from the insurance companies, and usually averages just a few weeks in most cases. Outpatient services vary widely in duration and may last a few weeks to several months. Again, insurance benefits may play a significant role in determining the duration of these services.

Overall, the duration of rehabilitation services after a stroke varies from a few weeks to as long as six months or even longer in selected cases. It is important to recognize that neurological function and ability to perform daily tasks can and often do continue to improve after the completion of formal rehabilitation services. As the rehabilitation program progresses, the stroke survivor and his family need to accept increasing responsibility for performing exercises at home without the direct presence of a rehabilitation therapist. This will allow for a smooth transition once formal services end and, perhaps more important, will help the stroke survivor attain the highest degree of function achievable. Ultimately, the rehabilitation team is only a guide. The real work is always done by the stroke survivor himself.

7

Stroke in the Young and the Old

Gertrude is an eighty-nine-year-old woman who suddenly develops slurred speech and loss of balance. She is admitted to a community hospital near her home, where she is diagnosed with a stroke. Since the death of her husband ten years ago, she has lived alone and maintained an active lifestyle. She was driving until six months ago, when she was forced to stop because of macular degeneration, a disorder that causes progressive visual loss. The case manager at the hospital is encouraging her to receive her rehabilitation at a nearby skilled nursing facility (SNF). She tells Gertrude's daughter it is likely that she will remain in the long-term care program at the same facility. The daughter is concerned that the case manager's recommendation to send her mother to a skilled nursing facility is based only on her age. Is this the best choice for Gertrude? Is she too old for more intensive rehabilitation?

Stroke in the Elderly

Stroke can affect people throughout life, though it is most common among older individuals. The risk of stroke rises steadily as we age and doubles each decade after age fifty. The issues stroke survivors face vary depending on their age.

Good recoveries from stroke can also occur at any age. As a general rule of thumb, however, rehabilitation becomes more difficult as people age; or, as someone once put it, "Old age isn't for sissies." Anti-elder bias, sometimes referred to as "ageism," is widely prevalent throughout our society and is surprisingly common in the medical world. Medical or surgical treatments, such as carotid artery surgery to prevent another stroke, or the use of Coumadin (warfarin) for similar purposes, should not be automatically excluded because of age alone. The risks of certain treatments may rise with age, but each person needs to be evaluated as an individual rather than on the basis of age.

Similarly, no older person should be denied the benefits of rehabilitation simply because of her age. I have cared for a number of patients in their nineties who have made good recoveries after stroke. When evaluating the effects of stroke on the elderly, it is essential to have an accurate understanding of the prestroke level of function. Frequently an older person who has had gradually declining abilities for some time will manage to continue independent functioning in the home environment. When even a minor stroke occurs, it may bring into full view just how much difficulty the older person was having before the illness. In such cases the stroke may seem to have a disproportionate effect on the person's independence.

Gertrude's daughter, after visiting the SNF, advocates for a more aggressive rehabilitation program with a goal of Gertrude's eventual return to the community. After a three-week stay at a rehabilitation hospital near the daughter's home, Gertrude moves in with her daughter. The daughter sets up a first-floor apartment for her mother, and Gertrude is able to manage with only minor assistance. Both report that they are happy with the living arrangements.

Cognitive flexibility, the ability to learn new ways of thinking and problem solving, may decline in advanced age, even when more established thinking abilities do not show decline. Since dealing with the effects of a stroke can involve learning many new approaches to basic daily tasks, an older person may have more trouble with this aspect of rehabilitation than a younger person would.

Aging is associated with a decrease in muscle mass and strength, which appears to contribute to the loss of reserve strength. For example, a young person with weakness after a stroke may have enough strength on his unaffected side to stand easily on his "good" leg. An older person may have had trouble rising from a low surface even before a stroke, and require considerable assistance to stand even with the same neurological limitations as the younger person. Compounding this reduced strength is the frequent presence of arthritis in the elderly, as well as other unrelated medical conditions such as heart disease, vision and hearing loss, and so on.

Many older individuals experience an increase in fatigueability, a symptom that can be exacerbated after stroke. This increased fatigue may make rehabilitation slower than usual but should not lead to discontinuation of the effort. All these concerns need to be kept in perspective—many older stroke survivors have excellent recoveries after stroke, despite these challenges.

Elderly stroke survivors may have less support available at home than younger patients to help them manage after a stroke. It is not uncommon for older people to have lost a spouse or have a spouse who is disabled and requires assistance, limiting the stroke survivor's options for living arrangements. Complicating this situation is the fact that many families today are members of the "sandwich" generation, with children to care for at home as well as a disabled parent, not to mention a full-time job.

Older people are generally more sensitive to the side effects of medications, and this may be amplified by the effects of a stroke. Medications that are sedating may be poorly tolerated even in lower doses in the elderly. The stroke survivor and her family should carefully discuss with the prescribing physician the risks and benefits of any new medication, as well as any potential side effects.

As Gertrude's case shows, however, advanced age does not preclude successful rehabilitation. There are certainly challenges in rehabilitation of elderly stroke survivors, but with support from the family and dedicated healthcare professionals, many older individuals are able to return to the community after a stroke.

For patients who cannot return home or go to live with family, an assisted living facility or nursing home may be necessary. Is such cases, it is essential for family members to face up to the new reality in order to maximize the quality of life for the stroke survivor.

Stroke in Young Adults

Becky is a twenty-four-year-old graduate student pursuing her Ph.D. in molecular biology when she suddenly develops a stroke due to a previously asymptomatic vascular malformation (AVM) in her brain. She experiences right-sided weakness and aphasia. Her family flies in to support her during her hospitalization and rehabilitation. Afterward, she can walk with a cane but still has minimal movement in her right hand, as well as trouble finding the words she wishes to use. In addition to the direct effects of the stroke, Becky has been quite depressed and is pessimistic about returning to school.

Her boyfriend, who is also a graduate student, has tried to be supportive through her illness but is struggling with mixed feelings of commitment to Becky and concerns regarding the future of their relationship. Becky's parents, who have no other children, are trying to be as helpful and supportive as possible, but Becky finds their attention overwhelming at times. She feels they are treating her like a child again. How can Becky and her family work together to help her recover?

Becky's story points out some of the unique problems confronting young people with stroke. While everyone's situation is different, some common themes emerge among young stroke survivors. Work and school issues tend to be much more prominent in this population than in those who are retired or near retirement. For this reason, treatment of stroke in young people must include a detailed assessment of work abilities, as well as focused efforts to prepare the patient for return to work or school. Neuropsychological evaluation may be particularly useful, since it provides a very detailed and thorough assessment of cognitive (thinking) and language abilities. Vocational counseling is another important resource and can help survivors obtain job coaching or retraining as appropriate.

The brain's ability to recover from a stroke is greater in young adults than in older individuals. Since many medical professionals are most accustomed to the recovery process in older people with stroke (who form the vast majority of stroke survivors), they must be careful not to underestimate the potential for recovery in a young adult. If the physician, rehabilitation therapist, or insurance company appears to be prematurely concluding that a young stroke survivor has reached a plateau in her recovery, family members may need to actively advocate on her behalf. Young stroke survivors may require longer, more intensive rehabilitation than their elderly counterparts to achieve their maximal potential for recovery after stroke.

Family issues vary dramatically for stroke survivors depending on their age. Recovery may involve parents, children, boyfriends, domestic partners, spouses, or others. For someone just emerging into adulthood, like Becky, the regression toward old roles can be particularly stressful. The parents of a person who has a stroke in her thirties or forties may become involved in their child's life in a way they never anticipated or planned for. Spouses may find themselves with a disabled partner; significant others or domestic partners may find themselves questioning the degree of commitment they have made to someone who has now changed and, in some cases, become dependent on others for assistance.

As is evident from this discussion, the definition of "young" is always a moving target and may reflect life roles more than actual chronological age. Whatever the age, stroke is a stressful event. In order to maximize a survivor's recovery, family members must discuss their loved one's unique issues with the rehabilitation team. Together they can develop a plan to work toward shared goals.

Stroke in Children

Stroke is usually thought of as a disease of older adults, but it can occur at any age. In fact, stroke can even occur before birth. Children's ability to recover from a stroke differs substantially from adults', as does the impact that stroke has on their lives and development. During childhood the brain is still developing and so retains greater "plasticity" (flexibility of structure and function) than the adult brain. For this reason children with stroke are able to show substantial improvements that may far exceed the ability of adult survivors. Nonetheless, there are limits to the brain's ability to compensate for injury, and thus child survivors face many of the same issues as adults as they learn to live with a disability. It is also important to understand that this increased ability of the brain to cope with injury doesn't begin and end on a neat schedule; rather, it exists as a continuum, with the greatest plasticity as a young child, and gradual reduction of this plasticity over a lifetime.

Rehabilitation for young children differs in another key respect from rehabilitation among adults. Whereas adults are typically relearning activities they could perform prior to stroke, many children with stroke are acquiring abilities for the first time. Some refer to this process of helping children acquire new skills as "habilitation" rather than as "rehabilitation," to emphasize that these skills are not being reacquired but rather are being learned for the first time.

A thorough discussion of the impact of stroke on children is beyond the scope of this book. For more information, see the resources listed in the Appendix.

8

Impact on Marriage and Relationships

Peter and Lilly have been married for thirty years and have raised two children who are now grown and living in another state. Peter's career as a successful executive in a Fortune 500 company creates substantial demands on his life even when he's not in the office. Lilly returned to work as a social worker after their children were grown. She has played an important role in Peter's professional life as a spouse and hostess and has provided him with significant emotional support. Peter has always been very loving to Lilly but has to a large extent depended on her to manage their family and social life. Friends and business associates have long admired their successful relationship.

Their marriage is put to the test by Lilly's sudden stroke. She experiences left-sided weakness, cognitive difficulties, and a loss of social skills. At first Peter is unable to accept the changes in Lilly, and devotes his energies to finding her "the best" treatment, which he believes will return her to her previous function. Gradually he comes to accept that while Lilly has improved significantly, she will have some permanent disability. He arranges twenty-four-hour assistance for Lilly at their home and is largely able to resume his prior work schedule. Fortunately, he is able to curtail his work-related travel schedule and is home with Lilly every evening. Peter remains frustrated by his new situation, however. He confides in a close friend that even though his wife is home, he "misses the old Lilly." He feels that he no longer has the emotional support he has always counted on, and has lost his primary confidante and best friend. Lilly seems largely unaware of the changes in their relationship, though she sometimes unexpectedly accuses Peter of no longer loving her. How can Peter and Lilly adapt to the changes in their relationship?

Stroke does not just affect the stroke survivor; it affects all those around him. Usually the spouse is the person most directly impacted. In cases of disabling stroke, a spouse who was once a strong partner may suddenly be recast in a more dependent role. A spouse who formerly was a source of support and nurture now may not only be unable to provide this support, but may require nurture himself.

Peter and Lilly's situation is not uncommon. There is no "going back" after a stroke, and understanding the changes in the relationship is a difficult but important step in moving forward. A healthy spouse may find that her husband is no longer able to meet her emotional needs after a stroke. By turning to friends and family for support she may actually help remove some of the pressure from the marriage and establish a new equilibrium. In Peter's case, his relationship with his brother is a major source of strength for him. Whereas he once turned to his wife for advice about his career, he now learns to rely on his brother.

Providing care to a spouse after a stroke creates multiple challenges for a relationship. The time requirements of providing assistance or supervision can be daunting in their own right. This is particularly true if the healthy spouse is still working or if children are still at home. Many people struggle with conflicting demands between family responsibilities and work even without contending with the aftereffects of a stroke. Sometimes a stroke can feel like the straw that broke the camel's back.

The physical demands of caregiving can also be substantial, to the point of becoming unmanageable. An older spouse may have medical problems of his own that interfere with his ability to provide assistance to his wife.

Spouses are generally accustomed to a substantial degree of intimacy, but the care needs after a stroke may require accepting new roles and breaking down former barriers of privacy. Helping a spouse with toileting, for example, may cause emotional discomfort for some couples. Injecting a spouse with insulin may be difficult emotionally for some individuals. Fortunately, we are all often more capable of adapting to new situations than we give ourselves credit for. Most spouses can meet the challenge of providing care to a partner in ways they never felt possible. In cases where healthy spouses simply cannot manage on their own, other resources, such as home health aides or personal-care attendants, can be called upon to reduce the burden to a manageable level.

Accepting assistance from anyone can be very difficult for some stroke survivors, and even more so if this assistance is being provided by a spouse. A stroke survivor who has always been highly independent or is used to being the dominant partner in the marriage will often struggle with her newly dependent role. Identifying this challenge is the first step in addressing it. Lifelong habits and behaviors can be difficult to change, so it is essential for both spouses to work together to reach a new arrangement.

Communication between spouses is essential after stroke. This is easiest when cognitive abilities and language are spared by a stroke, but even when these areas have been affected, the healthy spouse needs to make certain that a dialogue continues. Spending time discussing the changes in their lives and marital roles may be helpful to both members of the marriage. Many couples feel better simply by airing the emotional issues that they face individually and together. Marital counseling may be useful for couples who find it difficult to work through these issues on their own.

Some marriages end in divorce after stroke. Sometimes stroke represents the final stressor for a marriage that was already in trouble before the stroke. In other cases, the healthy spouse is unable to accept her partner's altered behavior and abilities. More commonly, stroke induces a review of priorities. Many couples find that dealing with a major life stressor such as stroke can actually strengthen their relationship.

Physical closeness in the form of hugging, cuddling, and touching may be a source of strength in a marriage after a stroke. Sex can also be a shared pleasure that continues to be a significant support for the marriage, though some adaptations to physical disability imposed by the stroke may be necessary.

Sex

Frank is a fifty-nine-year-old married insurance salesman with diabetes and hypertension. He wakes one morning to find that he cannot stand and is weak on his left side. Though he makes a relatively rapid and substantial recovery from his stroke, he develops depression and is given fluoxetine (Prozac) by his physician. He seems to be doing well when he comes to his primary care doctor for a visit. As he is leaving the exam room, however, he asks the physician if he would be able to take Viagra (sildenafil). After his physician has him return to the room and discuss the issue further, it becomes clear that Frank was having difficulty maintaining erections even before his stroke, and has had increased difficulties since his stroke. He also reports a loss of libido (sex drive). Lastly, he reports that both he and his wife are worried about precipitating another stroke during sex. Should Frank and his wife worry that sex might cause another stroke? If not, are his sexual problems treatable? What is causing these symptoms?

Sex plays an important role in marriage and long-term relationships beyond its direct physical pleasures. Owing to the serious and often disabling nature of stroke, healthcare practitioners often neglect the topic of sexuality after stroke. Stroke survivors themselves may be embarrassed to raise the issue, or they may assume that their disability precludes resumption of sexual activity. Despite the apparent public preoccupation with sexuality, it is often given insufficient attention in the context of illness such as stroke.

Sexual function may be negatively impacted by a number of aspects of stroke, and it may be difficult in some cases to determine what the primary limiting factors are. Loss of sensation can occur with stroke, directly impacting sexual function in both men and women. The weakness and abnormal muscle tone that accompany stroke can directly interfere with the mechanics of intercourse. Couples may find it helpful to explore alternative positions in which the stroke-affected partner can participate in sex with fewer physical challenges. For example, intercourse may be easier for both people if the affected partner lies on his or her back during intercourse.

Although many couples find it difficult to talk about sex, discussing the challenges faced with a physician or nurse can be enormously helpful. For example, the abnormal muscle spasms sometimes triggered by sex can be controlled with medications in many cases.

Medication side effects are quite common and can lead to reduced libido, arousal, or orgasm in men and women. Men may experience erectile dysfunction (impotence or inability to achieve an erection) or ejaculatory dysfunction. Many antihypertensive medications are known to cause erectile dysfunction in some men and may contribute to sexual dysfunction in women as well, with beta-blockers such as propanolol (Inderal) a particularly common culprit. Antidepressant medications can cause loss of interest in sex as well as impotence or delayed orgasm in some cases.

Antidepressants in the Prozac family, such as Celexa (citalopram), Zoloft (sertraline), and Paxil (paroxetine), are particularly common causes of sexual dysfunction.

Common medical conditions, such as diabetes, that are risk factors for stroke can themselves affect sexual functioning. In some cases, such as Frank's, these other conditions affect sexual function before a stroke to some extent, and then become more symptomatic in combination with the stroke itself. Viagra and related medications can be quite effective in the appropriate circumstances in helping restore sexual function in men, and perhaps in some women as well. Because of the risk of interaction with other medications and medical issues, these medications should be obtained and used only after discussion with a physician, and then taken only as prescribed.

For men affected by erectile dysfunction who are unable to use medications because of medical contraindications, or for whom these medications are ineffective, other options exist to facilitate resumption of sexual activity. These include injections of medications or the use of a suction device to produce an erection, or the use of surgical penile implants in appropriate cases. Consultation with a urologist specializing in erectile dysfunction is advisable.

Sexual dysfunction in women after stroke is less well studied and understood than sexual dysfunction in men. There are also fewer established treatments for women experiencing sexual dysfunction after a stroke. Women should consult a urologist or gynecologist specializing in sexual dysfunction if review of medications and other initial efforts are unsuccessful.

Psychological factors play a key role in many cases of sexual dysfunction after illness. Many stroke survivors feel they are less sexually attractive than before the stroke. Healthy partners can help resolve the problem by confirming that they are still attracted to the stroke survivor and truly wish to resume their prior sexual relationship. Fears of precipitating another stroke or other medical complications are common among both stroke survivors and their partners, but are generally unfounded. There is no evidence that sexual activity is likely to precipitate a stroke. Nonetheless, before leaving the hospital patients should confirm with their physician that it is safe to resume sex (with appropriate contraception when needed).

Fatigue is common after stroke, and some individuals may also experience changes in their libido. Rather than waiting to have sex until going to bed at night, some couples find that having sex earlier in the day is more practical, especially when excessive fatigue is an issue. Anxiety may interfere with sex initially, but it typically resolves as a couple becomes reacquainted with each other.

Spouses whose partners require significant help with daily activities sometimes find it hard to switch out of the caregiver role. Helping their significant other get dressed, use the bathroom, and so on may make it difficult for the caregiving spouse (or affected partner) to resume a more romantic role. As with many of the issues surrounding sexual activity after a stroke, understanding and patience are important steps in surmounting this problem. Caregiver support groups provide a helpful forum for discussing with others in the same situation the emotional consequences of providing care for a stroke survivor.

Aphasia can affect the social context for sex, including making it difficult for the stroke survivor to let his partner know when he is interested in sex. While these communication difficulties can be overcome (sex is, after all, a nonverbal form of communication to some extent), the inability to have the verbal interchange that leads up to sex can be awkward at first. Working through this together can help partners establish new and effective ways of communicating about a very important issue.

Cognitive or behavioral changes in the stroke survivor may impact a healthy spouse's interest in sex. Sexual attraction to a partner is based on both physical and emotional interactions. Some unaffected partners may no longer feel sexually attracted to a stroke survivor whose behavior has changed, or whose ability to interact verbally has been diminished. In other cases, the healthy partner may feel that it is wrong to have sex with a partner who is cognitively impaired. The healthy partner must recognize these feelings in order to deal with them constructively. Remembering that sex is mutually enjoyable and a source of pleasure for the stroke survivor may help the healthy partner overcome initial reservations about resumption of sexual activity.

Physical intimacy in a relationship consists of much more than sex. Many couples find that they can reestablish a physical bond by hugging, cuddling, caressing, and kissing. Stroke survivors and their partners should not let the stroke and its residual effects interfere with these important and mutually beneficial physical affections.

Contraception

With resumption of sex, the need for contraception may exist for many younger stroke survivors. An unplanned pregnancy after a stroke can be emotionally challenging and in some cases even medically hazardous. For this reason, reliable and safe contraception is especially important after stroke.

Oral contraceptives ("the pill") are one of the most reliable and convenient forms of birth control, but they may be problematic for women after a stroke. In some cases, oral contraceptives may actually increase the risk of a recurrent stroke and may be inadvisable medically. Women should discuss the risks and benefits of using oral contraceptives with a physician before considering this form of contraception after stroke.

Barrier methods of contraception, such as condoms or a diaphragm, are generally quite safe after stroke. Their reliability depends in part on proper use. Some of these methods, such as contraceptive foams, are significantly less reliable and should probably be avoided in cases where pregnancy needs to be scrupulously avoided.

Intrauterine devices (IUDs) are a highly effective form of contraception that may be particularly appropriate for young women after a stroke. IUDs have unfortunately been stigmatized by their association with pelvic infection and infertility in young women who are not in long-term monogamous relationships. An IUD may be an excellent choice for a woman with a stroke who has completed her family and is in a stable monogamous relationship. Women considering this form of birth control should discuss the pros and cons with a gynecologist.

All sexually active women of childbearing age should discuss contraception with their primary care or other treating physician. Unfortunately, many physicians fail to raise this issue with their patients after stroke, and miscommunication is common.

Pregnancy after Stroke

Juanita is a thirty-four-year-old nurse who was married for three years at the time of her stroke and has recently completed her rehabilitation program. She has always wanted a family and is concerned that her "biological clock is ticking." She asks her physician, "Is it safe for me to become pregnant?

What difficulties should I expect during pregnancy, delivery, and raising my child?"

Juanita's situation presents complex questions, and the answers vary substantially from person to person. For many young women after stroke, having children can be every bit as satisfying and successful as for any other mother. For others, however, pregnancy may be hazardous and inadvisable. Issues that need to be considered when contemplating a pregnancy after stroke include the severity of remaining disability, the cause and type of stroke, and any ongoing medical issues. Some medications used after stroke, such as certain antiseizure medications or Coumadin (warfarin), can be dangerous for an unborn child and can cause fetal malformations. Pregnancy and vaginal delivery may be risky for a woman with an arteriovenous malformation (AVM).

For individuals with medical contraindications to pregnancy, adoption may be a viable alternative. Assisted reproduction techniques, such as arranging for a surrogate mother to carry a pregnancy for the stroke survivor and her husband, may be an option in special cases.

Given the complexity of the issues surrounding pregnancy after stroke, consultation with both a neurologist and an obstetrician/gynecologist (ob/gyn) specializing in high-risk pregnancies is often helpful. A team approach may be required to provide full consideration of the issues involved and develop a plan that is safe for mother and child, in addition to meeting the personal goals of the woman and her partner.

For men affected by stroke, the issues of parenting are not directly medical (except in cases of sexual dysfunction) but focus instead on the impact of any residual disability on parenting and the marital relationship. Parenting can present a substantial stress for any couple; a couple coping with the aftermath of a stroke needs to consider their decision thoughtfully. There is no denying the incredible pleasure that parenting can provide, however, and stroke survivors are as entitled as anyone else to partake in this most sublime experience.

9

Impact on Children and Family

Sam, forty-five, is an active, successful entrepreneur with his own small business as a broker in computer memory chips. Although he has several employees, the business relies heavily on his knowledge of the market for these chips, and he works long hours. His wife, Lisa, is a forty-year-old grade school teacher who recently returned to work after taking several years off to raise their two young children, Ashley and Michael. Ashley is now nine and Michael is six. Both are performing well at school. Sam also has an eighteen-year-old son, Chris, from a previous marriage, who is a freshman in college in another state. Sam's life changes dramatically after he sustains a stroke affecting the left side of his brain, resulting in aphasia and severe right-sided weakness. His family's life has also been changed in ways they are only beginning to understand. His wife is trying to figure out what the future holds for them. Will Sam ever be able to go back to work? If not, will she need to be at home with Sam? If so, how will they support themselves? What will happen to his business? How will the children react to their father's disability?

Sam's family is faced with an almost unimaginable change; they will gradually need to develop a new lifestyle that will incorporate the effects of Sam's stroke. Each family experiences different challenges and has different resources to help them cope. There is no blueprint that works for every family, but there are certain common themes that can help loved ones deal with the life-altering changes stroke can cause.

Taking One Step at a Time

The enormity of the challenges posed by stroke, particularly in a situation like Sam's, requires a staged approach. Lisa will not be able to solve all the problems she faces immediately. After the initial whirlwind of the acute hospital stay is over, Sam is transferred to a rehabilitation hospital. The rehabilitation hospital staff estimate that Sam will be at the facility for approximately four to five weeks, during which time Lisa can begin to sort out certain issues. Some concerns, like determining how to pay for their children's college educations, will simply have to wait until more immediate issues are addressed.

Lisa's mother-in-law (Sam's mother), who is retired and in good health, offers to stay with Lisa while Sam is still in the hospital. Accepting help from friends and family may be hard in a society that prizes independence, but assistance from extended family can be invaluable in helping a family cope with the impact of a stroke. Sam's mother helps out with his two young children, allowing Lisa to concentrate on supporting Sam during his rehabilitation.

Because of the nature of Sam's business, Lisa must next make some quick decisions regarding the likelihood of his returning to work. The business is very time-sensitive and not easily restarted after a prolonged closure. Lisa is understandably concerned that Sam will be unable to return to his duties, and she discusses his prognosis with his physician. While Sam is only two weeks out from his stroke, he remains severely aphasic, and the CT scans and MRIs confirm that the stroke has severely damaged the speech centers in his brain. Although his ultimate prognosis remains uncertain, it is clear that he will be disabled for many months at a minimum, and the company cannot manage without him for that long. The good news is that Sam recently took out a long-term disability insurance policy, which should provide enough money for the family to pay its bills, though much less than they were accustomed to having. Lisa puts together a plan to sell the business before the clients evaporate, though she finds this a painful experience, knowing how hard her husband worked to build the business.

The Children

Sam's three children face different issues in coping with the effects of the stroke. His eldest son, Chris, outwardly appears to have the easiest time accepting the stroke and its aftereffects. Inwardly he is angry and frustrated. He feels cheated because he has never had as much time with his father as he would have liked growing up. Now that his father has had a stroke, Chris doubts that he will ever have the opportunity to spend quality time with him. He wonders if he should take time off from college to spend with his father, even though his own mother and Lisa advise against this. He wonders how he will be able to concentrate on his studies, knowing that his father is in the hospital.

Lisa, supported by Chris's mother, tries to help Chris through this crisis. The two women advise Chris that he should spend as much time with his father as feels right to him, but reassure him that a good plan is in place to care for Sam in the hospital and at home. They remind Chris that Sam has always been supportive of Chris's educational efforts and would likely want him to continue his studies uninterrupted. While Chris ultimately decides to return to school and complete the semester, it is important to recognize that there is no universally correct approach in such situations. It may be an equally reasonable alternative for Chris to take a semester off from college to spend time with his father and family.

The two younger children are having trouble understanding what has happened to their father. They know that he is "sick," but they continue to ask when he will get better. Michael has begun having nightmares and is now sleeping with his mother. Ashley is afraid that her father will die, though she has not verbalized this concern. Coping with stroke can be particularly challenging for young children, but at the same time they are often more resilient than we think. Allowing the children to visit their father in the hospital will reassure them that he is still around. Having them draw pictures and get-well cards at home will give them a sense that they are helping their father recover from his illness. Encouraging them to express their fears verbally will help Lisa address their specific concerns and allay many of their fears.

Some degree of regression, when children appear to go backward developmentally, is common in younger children dealing with the trauma of a sick parent. This common response to stress in young children generally resolves on its own and should not be a source of concern unless it persists. Similarly, an increased need for emotional support and physical proximity (for example, wanting to sleep with a family member) is common, and adults should focus on providing the reassurance and emotional support needed, rather than on enforcing previous practices (such as requiring the children to sleep in their own beds). If these regressive behaviors continue for an excessive duration, family counseling may be helpful. Counseling is also useful for children who are expressing, either verbally or through their actions, excessive anxiety, agitation, or depression.

Returning Home

Despite the best efforts of the rehabilitation team and family to prepare for discharge home, readjustment is often very stressful. In cases like Sam's, where significant disability persists, the demands on caregivers are easily underestimated. This transition is a good time to "call in the reserves" and have an extra friend or family member stay over for the first few days or weeks.

Those caring for individuals with disabling stroke need to be certain that their own needs are not ignored. The stresses on caregivers can be enormous and may be sustained over many years. Scheduling time for the caregiver in the overall plan for tending to a disabled stroke survivor is critical to the long-term success of the plan. In Lisa's case, she is faced with the needs not only of her husband but also of her two young children. After taking a family leave to help get her husband settled at home, Lisa is planning to return to her teaching position. Work will help her meet the family's financial needs and maintain her own professional identity.

Sam returns home and begins an active program of home rehabilitation through the visiting nurse agency. After a few weeks, he transitions to a day rehabilitation program a few miles from his home. He is dropped off at 9 A.M. and picked up at 2 P.M. after having his physical, occupational, and speech therapy, as well as lunch and some social activities. His wife is gratified by his progress in rehabilitation but remains concerned about their future lifestyle. Sam is still unable to express himself well verbally, though he is able to speak in short, halting sentences and communicate to a limited extent. He is now walking well with a cane and rarely uses the wheelchair. He still has very limited movement in his arm. Lisa wonders how she will be able to return to work. Can her husband be by himself safely? How long should she ask her mother-in-law to stay with them? She feels bad that she has required so much help from

her mother-in-law and is concerned at the same time that she is not giving her children enough attention. How can she cope?

Young children face a special challenge when coping with a parent's
stroke. In Sam's case, the children are happy to have their father back at
home but are puzzled by the changes that have occurred. Why can't he
give them piggyback rides like he did before? Over time, children usually
adapt well to new circumstances caused by a stroke, but they may face
problems with social embarrassment related to their parent's disability.
Questions such as, "Why does your father talk funny?" or "Why can't
your father drive us to the movies?" may cause particular discomfort for
adolescent children and teenagers.

Some family activities may prove difficult for a parent after a stroke.
Depending on the nature of the stroke, the parent may have difficulty
helping with various aspects of homework or providing rides to activities.
Except in the most severe cases, stroke survivors usually retain substantial ability to provide emotional support and love, however, and this is often the most important and underappreciated parental role. As with
healthy parents, each person brings a variety of strengths and weak-
nesses to the challenges of parenthood, and can maximize effective-
ness by recognizing these abilities and limitations. Expanding the role of
other relatives, such as uncles, aunts, or grandparents, may enrich a
child's life in any family, and provide particular support in a family where
one parent has had a stroke.

Parents with stroke may find that their impaired abilities place them at
a disadvantage in providing discipline and guidance during the teenage
years, when children commonly test and question authority. Recognizing this difficulty early on may allow the healthy parent to intervene in a
timely manner. Family counseling may prove useful in some cases to
bring these issues into open discussion.

Mildred, age seventy-nine, and Max, age eighty, were enjoying their later
years together and recently celebrated their fiftieth wedding anniversary.
A few days after their anniversary party, Max suddenly develops garbled
speech, becomes confused, and can't move his right side. Despite the efforts to rehabilitate Max, he remains unable to walk and requires considerable help to move from the bed to the wheelchair or to the bathroom.

Mildred has osteoporosis and has previously had wrist and hip fractures, leaving her physically frail. One of their sons is in the army, and the other is a truck driver who lives on the opposite coast. Both are supportive but cannot provide significant help to their parents. Mildred would like to take Max home, but she feels overwhelmed by his care needs. His discharge date from the rehabilitation unit nears, and she can't decide what to do. Should Mildred have Max transferred to a nursing home?

If Mildred and Max were fortunate enough to have considerable financial resources, they might be able to consider hiring live-in, twenty-four-hour-a-day help. As with most people, however, this option is beyond their means. Instead, Mildred is faced with the difficult decision of placing Max in a nursing home. For a variety of reasons, ranging from American family structures to cultural values and financial considerations, a nursing home may be the only reasonable option in some cases after stroke. In such situations the loved one burdened with this decision needs other family members to support her and provide reassurance that she did the best she could in a situation with few options. Although most people prefer to live at home, sometimes it just isn't possible given the available resources.

Key considerations in Max's case are to ensure that the nursing home selected provides high-quality care in a pleasant, stimulating environment, and that Mildred is able to spend as much time with Max as she likes. Transportation issues are often critical for elderly spouses, who may not be able to drive to visit. Some view nursing homes as warehouses for the elderly or anterooms to the end of life. The extent to which these stereotypes are true depends in part on the attitudes and involvement of family members, who can help keep a resident of a nursing home connected socially and stimulated mentally.

Nursing homes are more complex organizations than they once were, and many now include short-term rehabilitation units that are focused on returning people home. Such units are not appropriate for all individuals, of course. Those who do receive their rehabilitation in this type of unit should be assured that discharge home remains the plan, rather than long-term residency in the nursing home. Often such units provide a middle road for stroke survivors who are not yet ready to return home, but for whom the possibility of home discharge remains viable.

10

Return to Work and Leisure Activities

Nat is a fifty-two-year-old firefighter in a busy urban community. He has worked hard to improve his skills and has advanced through the ranks to captain of a fire-fighting squad. He suddenly develops a stroke while on a vacation cruise and is airlifted off the ship to a nearby hospital. After completing his rehabilitation, he is left with left-hand clumsiness but otherwise has had a full recovery. As someone who loves his work, he is determined to return to fire-fighting duties. Can Nat resume work as a firefighter? If not, what can he do instead?

Nat embarks on an aggressive program of vocational rehabilitation. In spite of his best efforts, however, he finds that many emergency duties (for example, managing a fire hose, turning valves) require two highly functional hands. He concludes that he cannot safely resume his prior duties. He retrains as an arson inspector and finds employment that uses his skills and experience in this area.

Many people think of work as merely a way to obtain financial resources, and for some people work provides little else. More commonly, however, work plays multiple roles in our lives, helping to define who we are, how we view ourselves, and how we are viewed by those around us. It helps us develop unique areas of expertise, provides a focus for our efforts to improve ourselves, and contributes to a feeling of productivity and value to society. Thus for most people losing the ability to work has broad emotional ramifications beyond the obvious loss of wages.

These same issues are just as relevant for homemakers and volunteers as they are for those who work for salaries outside the home. The sudden loss of or dramatic change in these roles poses a major challenge to many people.

Age is often a factor in whether a stroke survivor decides to return to work. Stroke is most common among older individuals, and thus the majority of stroke survivors are retired at the time of their stroke. For another substantial group of survivors, stroke occurs as they are nearing retirement, and they do not seriously consider returning to work. For younger people, however, return to work is frequently a key issue and helps define their recovery from stroke.

Many factors influence the ability to return to work after a stroke. These include the motivation of the individual, the direct effects of the stroke, the type of work previously performed, and the extent of support the employer provides.

Motivation is key when determining if and when someone should rejoin the workforce. Except in the mildest cases, stroke adds to the challenges that work normally presents. Someone who is committed to her employment can often overcome these challenges. By contrast, someone who is indifferent to her work, or even dislikes it, may find these obstacles insurmountable. In some cases, even when the prior work was enjoyable, a stroke can cause someone to review priorities and goals for the future, resulting in a decision to change career goals or jobs. Someone who is financially secure may decide to devote her efforts to volunteer or advocacy work rather than returning to her earlier position. We should not automatically assume that returning to work is a goal for a stroke survivor; rather, healthcare professionals and family members should sit down and discuss with the patient what his specific goals are.

Stroke can cause a broad range of physical, emotional, cognitive, and communication problems. The unique difficulties faced by each person after a stroke need to be considered in the context of the person's specific work, rather than in general terms. Nat's case demonstrates the role of job duties in determining whether someone can return to a specific job after a stroke. Certain jobs, such as a plumber, electrician, or surgeon, require a high degree of bimanual dexterity, and even a moderate loss of hand function can interfere with successful return to work. At the same time, each of these fields may also include related work, such as teaching, or working as an electrical inspector, that may allow someone with reduced motor abilities to return to work in a different capacity.

Loss of cognitive or speech abilities is often the hardest area to overcome in return to work. As with jobs involving manual dexterity, jobs requiring high levels of cognitive or linguistic work may become problematic with even relatively mild degrees of disability. For someone whose work requires a high degree of spatial awareness and attention, such as a taxi driver or an air traffic controller, even mild deficits in these areas might be problematic, whereas they might not pose a problem for someone who works in sales. A lawyer, physician, or engineer may experience difficulty working with a mild cognitive impairment that would not interfere with less demanding professions. A careful analysis of job duties and frank assessment of retained abilities on the part of the stroke survivor can help determine if return to work is realistic in these cases. A neuropsychology assessment is often invaluable in helping a survivor assess her strengths and limitations after a stroke. Equally important, the person with stroke should define the specific job requirements necessary for her successful return to work. By identifying areas of the job that may pose particular difficulty, she can prepare herself early on for any problems that might arise.

The willingness of employers to modify work duties is another important factor in return to work. Attitudes toward working with a disability have gradually become more enlightened in the United States, but prejudice and misinformation are still common. Legal protections are now available for individuals with disabilities who are seeking to return to work. The Americans with Disabilities Act (ADA) prohibits employers from discriminating against individuals with disabilities, and requires them to make reasonable accommodations in the workplace to facilitate the employment or continued employment of disabled workers. The U.S. Department of Justice provides information on its web page and hotline regarding the protections provided by this law (see the Appendix).

Many people fall in a gray area, where successful return to work is uncertain and hard to predict reliably. Assuming that the employer is supportive, a staged approach is often helpful in these cases. The stroke survivor should provide the rehabilitation team with information regarding the nature of the work and the anticipated job tasks so they can establish specific goals and milestones in the rehabilitation program to prepare for return to work. This information will also allow the rehabilitation team to provide feedback regarding their assessments of readiness for return to work. Ideally, patients should help the team incorporate representative work tasks in the rehabilitation therapy program (for example, practicing a computer task, reviewing a budget, or working with a specific set of tools). These tasks may be practiced with an occupational or speech therapist, depending on the nature of the work. This collaboration between therapist and patient allows treatment to be directed to the specific areas of greatest importance to the stroke survivor in her return to work.

Vocational counseling plays a key role in return to work for individuals with significant disability after stroke. State-sponsored vocational rehabilitation programs are available in all fifty states and the District of Columbia to help with reentry into the workforce; they will also help people define alternative job options if a return to prior work is not possible. Stroke survivors planning a return to work should explore these resources early on rather than waiting until problems arise.

Depending on the circumstances, the stroke survivor may benefit from a visit to the workplace to refamiliarize himself with the work environment. Taking home some work (if practical) might help him reacquaint himself with specific job tasks outside the fast-paced work environment. If the tasks cannot be taken home, he might find it helpful to perform them at work in the presence of a job coach. This coach could be a supportive coworker, or, in some cases, an occupational or speech therapist, or other individual with the knowledge and skills to monitor and support the person's return to job tasks while at the same time providing emotional support if these prove too difficult.

If simulated work tasks are successful, initially returning to work part-time may be most appropriate. This gradual return can reduce the level of stress in the workplace and prevent coworkers or supervisors from assuming that the employee is ready to resume a full workload immediately. Many stroke survivors also experience substantially reduced endurance, which may become particularly evident when returning to a high-pressure work environment. Part-time work allows for rest periods and a more gradual increase in work responsibilities. An on-site job coach (typically a supportive coworker) may help provide extra support and monitor performance.

There are no firm rules regarding the timing of return to work after a stroke. While pressure to return promptly may be substantial, a premature return to work can do more harm than good. A person who attempts to return to work and is unsuccessful may be discouraged from attempting again. Moreover, the employer or supervisor may lose confidence in the abilities of the stroke survivor and hence be less supportive of a second attempt. Return to work should generally be delayed until the ability to perform activities of daily living and mobility has been maximized. Return to work in six to twelve months after a stroke is typical, though some individuals with a mild stroke can return sooner, and others will require more time.

Volunteer Work

Some individuals find they are unable or uninterested in returning to their prior employment but are nonetheless independent, energetic, and eager to be productive. While many people in this situation participate in vocational retraining, others choose to participate in the workplace as a volunteer. Volunteering affords many of the intangible rewards and satisfactions of work, as well as an opportunity for community service that is often lacking in traditional employment. Some use volunteer work as a bridge to returning to paid employment, whereas others find volunteering satisfying in its own right. I have had the pleasure of working with a number of my former patients who have chosen to volunteer their time in a rehabilitation hospital. As stroke survivors, they bring a unique perspective to more recent stroke patients with whom they interact, and can provide invaluable advice and emotional support. With health care (and other charitable organizations) chronically strapped for resources, volunteers can play an important role helping others with problems similar to or more severe than their own.

Managing Finances

For many people, the ability to manage their own financial affairs is an indicator of independence. Personal finance requires multiple skills, including the ability to read and write, perform math, and weigh the consequences of different courses of action. For individuals with cognitive or linguistic effects of stroke, managing personal finances can be problematic. At the same time, giving up these responsibilities can be emotionally traumatic.

Occupational and speech therapists often assess basic skills in this area, such as managing a checkbook. Patients should discuss the ability to manage basic finances with their therapist even before returning home from the hospital. In some cases, basic abilities may be preserved but questions still exist about higher-level tasks, such as managing investments. A neuropsychology evaluation can be very helpful in defining abilities and areas of concern; it can also help define which areas can be effectively managed by the stroke survivor and which cannot. When a loved one requires assistance in managing his or her financial affairs, a family member may find that obtaining a power of attorney is the best mechanism for providing this help.

Family members assuming primary responsibility for managing a stroke survivor's finances should make every effort to keep the stroke survivor as involved as possible in the decision-making. For example, a person who can no longer successfully manage a checkbook may still be able to select which charities she wishes to contribute to, or participate in discussions of estate planning. Supporting and encouraging this type of participation will help ensure that the stroke survivor's values and priorities are respected when making financial decisions, and support her feelings of self-worth and control over her life.

Driving and Transportation

For most Americans, driving is synonymous with freedom of movement. While more densely populated urban areas may provide a range of transportation options, driving is the only practical means for transportation throughout much of the United States. Return to driving can be a critical factor in return to work, shopping, entertainment, and social activities. For these reasons, return to driving is often a substantial concern of stroke survivors and one that many patients voice even prior to return home from the hospital.

Owing to the serious nature of stroke, most states require drivers to report this condition to the motor vehicle licensing agency and obtain a physician's report before driving again. If there is any doubt regarding driving safety after a stroke, the motor vehicle agency may require an examination and road test before allowing a stroke survivor to take the wheel. State regulations vary substantially, so it's a good idea to call your local agency before attempting to resume driving. It is also advisable for the stroke survivor to report the stroke to the automobile insurance company, since failure to do so may affect insurance coverage in the event of an accident.

Several aspects of stroke can affect driving ability, including visual losses, inattention or neglect syndromes, alexia (inability to read), weakness, reduced reaction time, cognitive deficits, and seizures. Loss of vision to the affected side (known as a visual field cut or deficit), even if not accompanied by reduced attention to the affected side, can impact driving ability. Regulations vary, but many states have minimum requirements for visual fields.

Driving requires managing a rapidly changing environment with unpredictable stimuli that can occur simultaneously. It requires the ability to sift through these stimuli rapidly and react promptly and accurately. For stroke survivors in whom attention to the affected side is impacted, or who have difficulty managing multiple stimuli simultaneously, driving is generally unsafe and best avoided. In cases where a mild difficulty exists in this area, many rehabilitation hospitals will provide "driving readiness" evaluations to measure perception and reaction time. These programs generally provide suggestions regarding adaptive equipment to assist the driver, and make recommendations regarding readiness to pursue an "on the road" driving test with the motor vehicle agency.

Weakness on one side does not generally preclude driving for someone without other major limitations caused by a stroke. Modifications to the car, including installation of a "spinner knob" device to allow one-handed steering (see Figure 10.1) and relocation of hand controls or pedals when needed can help make return to driving safe and practical. Certain driving schools with expertise in driving issues for people with disabilities can help a stroke survivor obtain the correct equipment and provide training in its use. Contact the Association of Driver Educators for the Disabled for more information (see Appendix). A road test with the state department of motor vehicles is generally required before someone using these automobile modifications may return to driving.

Seizures, though a relatively uncommon complication of stroke, have a substantial impact on return to driving. State laws governing driving

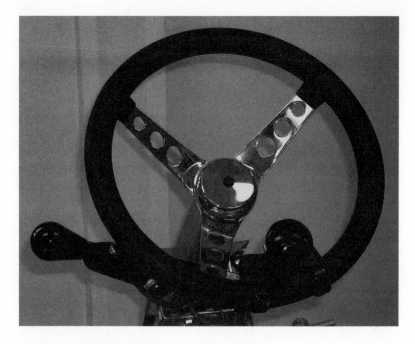

FIGURE 10.1   *Spinner device for one-handed steering.*

for individuals with a history of seizures vary and should be reviewed before returning to driving. Many require physician documentation that seizures have been controlled for an extended period prior to resuming driving. Some anticonvulsant (antiseizure) medications are also sedating and may affect driving ability as well.

Public transportation, including buses, trains, and subways, remains variably accessible to individuals with disabilities. Although wheelchair access continues to improve throughout cities in the United States, these systems are often challenging for someone with slowed mobility, balancing difficulties, and cognitive or perceptual problems to negotiate. Some metropolitan areas provide "paratransit" systems specifically designed for people with disabilities. Contact your local transportation authority for information on special transit accommodations in your area.

Air travel presents a challenge for people with stroke, though usually one that can be overcome. Medical prohibitions on air travel as a result of stroke are uncommon, though stroke survivors should consult their physicians before resuming air travel. Airlines will generally provide transportation assistance within the airport and onto the airplane. The actual airplane trip itself can be challenging, however, as minimal assistance is available during the flight. Airplane bathrooms are not accessible to anyone using a wheelchair, and any difficulty walking due to balance disturbances is compounded by the movement of the airplane in flight. With advance planning, however, most stroke survivors can return to air travel successfully.

Leisure Activities

Whereas return to work after stroke often receives considerable attention (especially for the young stroke survivor), return to leisure activities is frequently ignored. Immediately after a stroke, there is an appropriate focus on restoring the ability to perform basic daily tasks, such as dressing, walking, and so on. Restoring independent living at home then occupies the attention of the stroke survivor and the family, followed by return to work (depending on the stroke survivor's age and disability). Where does leisure activity fit in?

Leisure should be recognized as an important goal of rehabilitation from the outset. Americans place a high value on leisure activities and devote considerable time and resources to their pursuit. These activities range from crossword puzzles, to travel, to woodworking, kayaking, and even television (indeed, for many, this is the single most important leisure activity!). Because of the struggles that may accompany even basic daily tasks, many people with disabling strokes assume that leisure activities they once enjoyed are no longer available to them; nor do they consider new activities that may provide enjoyment. The range of leisure activities that can and have been adapted for a variety of disabling conditions is nearly limitless. Indeed, it is hard to think of a leisure activity that hasn't been adapted for this purpose, though clearly some lend themselves more easily to modification than others. Many organizations throughout the country are devoted to these activities and can provide experience and encouragement for participants. Many individuals and their families find their own personal solutions to the challenges of leisure activities, often exercising considerable creativity in the process.

What follows is not intended to be a comprehensive list of leisure activities for people with disabilities after stroke; rather, it is a small sample of the range of activities available. All these activities have one quality in common—they require the initiative of the individual or her family to be accessed. Personal initiative is particularly important for leisure pursuits; the healthcare system is focused on the treatment of disease and, to a lesser extent, disability, but often falls short of introducing people to what many see as "non-essential" pursuits. I believe leisure activities are quite important for resumption of a full and satisfying life. More information about accessing such activities is provided in the Appendix.

Examples of adapted sports and outdoor activities available for people with disabilities include:

- Bicycling
- Camping and hiking
- Golfing
- Horseback riding (hippotherapy)
- Sailing
- Water sports (kayaking, windsurfing, and others)

Guidebooks are available for people traveling with disabilities, and some tour operators specialize in this area (see Appendix). Specialized tour operators will also provide medical assistance or supervision for individuals requiring these services. With appropriate planning, there are few areas that are not accessible to stroke survivors with disabilities.

11

Weakness after Stroke

Peter is a fifty-nine-year-old car salesman with a history of high blood pressure and diabetes. Despite his physician's advice to exercise and lose weight, he has found it difficult to do so. He has had a few "spells" in which his left arm has felt "funny," but these have all gone away by themselves, and he has not mentioned them to his physician. One morning, he finds himself weak on the entire left side and is unable to stand up. After admission to the hospital, he is told that he has had a stroke that has severely affected his movement on the left side but has not caused any other damage. He is worried about his ability to return to work and is angry with himself for ignoring his transient ischemic attack (TIA) symptoms. He asks his physician, "When will my arm and leg start working again? Will I get all my strength back?"

Weakness is one of the most common problems after a stroke and a major contributor to disability. It is often the symptom that causes a person to seek medical attention for a stroke. Weakness generally occurs on the side of the body opposite the side of the brain affected by a stroke.

Weakness can result from stroke in several different locations in the brain. It may be the only stroke symptom in some cases, or it may occur with other problems, such as sensory loss or aphasia. While often referred to as "weakness," this symptom is more accurately described as loss of motor control (the ability to control and coordinate movements). Weakness resulting from stroke rarely occurs without a substantial loss of the ability to control and coordinate movements. Some individuals may have relative preservation of strength, with their primary problem consisting of loss of motor control and coordination. For example, a stroke survivor may be able to squeeze an object tightly with his hand (strength) but be unable to open the hand or move the fingers individually (control). Although significant weakness and loss of motor control often persist after a stroke, substantial recovery of movement may occur with appropriate rehabilitation.

Arm versus Leg

In the most common pattern of weakness after stroke, the arm is affected more than the leg, and the hand is the most severely impaired body part of all. There are several reasons for this pattern. First is the anatomy of stroke. A substantial percentage of strokes occur as a result of a clot ("embolus") lodging in an artery in the brain. The anatomy of the brain is such that the most direct path for a clot to travel is to the middle cerebral artery. This blood vessel supplies most of the primary motor control area of the brain. The area controlling the hand is located within the center of the region supplied by the middle cerebral artery; thus the function of the hand is usually severely affected by a blockage in this blood vessel (see Figure 4.3).

The second major factor affecting the functional recovery of the arm versus that of the leg relates to how the two limbs are used. The leg is normally used for relatively simple, repetitive movements. Someone who has very limited control of the leg but has enough leg stiffness to support his weight will often walk reasonably well after stroke. Conversely, the upper limb (and in particular, the hand) is called upon for much more specialized and demanding tasks. The hand needs extremely fine motor control for the broad range of tasks performed daily. Consider the gentle grasp required to hold a paper cup or a raw egg, the fine manipulation required to pick up a paper clip, or the firm grip needed to climb a ladder. Thus a stroke causing partial loss of control in the hand will have a larger impact on the ability to perform daily activities than a comparable stroke affecting the foot or leg.

Lastly, the complex and highly demanding motor functions of the hand require a substantial amount of brain "processing power" to direct them accurately. For this reason, the area of the brain devoted to the control of the arm and hand is quite a bit larger than the area devoted to the leg and foot (see Figure 4.2). Because they occupy a larger share of the brain, the areas controlling the upper limb are more likely to be affected by a stroke.

Reversed Pattern of Arm and Leg Weakness

Occasionally, a stroke will result from a blockage in the anterior cerebral artery rather than in the middle cerebral artery. Strokes resulting from this blockage tend to affect the leg more than the arm. Typically in these cases the leg is severely affected, the shoulder moderately weakened, and the hand minimally affected or not at all.

Exercise for Recovery

As discussed in Chapter 6, there is now strong evidence that the brain responds to activity (and in particular, exercise) with improved function. More research is still needed before we fully understand how much and which types of exercise provide the most benefit, but some basic principles are emerging. It is increasingly clear that exercise therapy improves the recovery of motor function and independence for people with weakness after stroke. Unfortunately, important questions remain regarding the best rehabilitation program after stroke. How much exercise therapy is the right amount after stroke? Is three hours of rehabilitation therapy each day (often used as a standard in rehabilitation hospitals) enough? More than enough? Too much for some people? How long should intensive therapy continue after stroke? What timing and intensity are appropriate for less intensive therapy afterward? Would maintenance therapy be beneficial if provided?

Despite the importance of these questions, definitive answers are not yet available. In the meantime, I believe that stroke survivors should be afforded the opportunity to do as much exercise and rehabilitation therapy as they can comfortably perform. The standard of three hours a day in a rehabilitation hospital appears reasonable, though some younger patients can do more, and some older or sicker individuals may not be capable of doing as much.

Is there such a thing as too much exercise, or starting too soon? The general rule of thumb is that the earlier rehabilitation is started, the better. There are limits to this approach, however, and some healthcare providers have questioned the safety of very aggressive rehabilitation in the first few days after a stroke. This concern is based on a study (conducted with animals, not people) which found that very aggressive exercise started immediately after a stroke actually worsened the damage caused by the stroke. Realistically speaking, however, no patients are likely to receive such intensive exercise programs so early after a stroke. In general, I recommend starting therapy programs as soon as a stroke survivor is medically stable enough to begin—typically within the first few days after a stroke. These exercise programs usually start gently and gradually increase in intensity as recovery progresses.

What type of exercise is most beneficial after stroke? Although there are many theories and substantial research in this area, no overall "philosophy" or approach to exercise has been found to be better than any other. Physical and occupational therapists receive training in one or more of these exercise techniques, such as neurodevelopmental technique (NDT, sometimes also known as Bobath, after its developer), Brunnstrom techniques, or proprioceptive neuromuscular facilitation (PNF). Most therapists in the United States have adopted an eclectic approach, whereby they take elements from multiple techniques to customize a therapy program for each patient. Most centers emphasize a "functionally oriented" approach for exercise therapy after stroke. This approach seeks to focus on the actual tasks that the stroke survivor will need to perform to achieve maximal independence. An example of this approach is practicing transfers from the wheelchair to the bed. This is an activity that will be very important for the non-ambulatory or partially ambulatory stroke survivor. Practicing the actual activity seems to be one of the best ways to learn how to do it independently. While this may seem obvious, some clinicians have argued in the past (and continue to argue, in some cases) that certain types or patterns of movements need to be mastered before the patient can train for a specific task, so that the correct "patterns" can be reestablished. This remains an interesting but unproven idea, and most therapists now focus directly on the challenge at hand.

During the process of rehabilitation, certain devices are often used to assist in reestablishing functional independence. These include braces for the lower leg, canes, and so on. Some stroke survivors are concerned that they may come to depend on these devices ("Doctor, I don't want to become dependent on a crutch") and not recover as much as they otherwise might. Practical considerations of returning home and being able to manage safely and independently argue strongly for use of these devices, however. I often point out to my patients that just because they have these devices and know how to use them does not mean they must be used all the time. Stroke survivors can (and often should) continue to practice without a cane or brace as much as they wish, as long as they have appropriate safety measures in place (for example, walking with someone for stability if needed). As recovery progresses, some people are able to discontinue or reduce the use of these devices, whereas others continue to require them to function independently.

After a few days in the acute care hospital, Peter is transferred to a rehabilitation hospital. During his three weeks at the rehabilitation hospital, he undergoes daily physical and occupational therapy for his left-sided weakness. He notes some gradual improvement in his leg but relatively little change in his arm. He still is unable to raise up his foot at the ankle and requires a plastic brace to help him walk. In the end, he is able to walk unassisted but needs a cane and a brace and has very limited use of his left arm.

New Treatment Approaches

Some new exercise techniques have generated considerable publicity and excitement within the field of stroke rehabilitation. These specialized and experimental techniques have thus far only been applied to specific aspects of stroke rehabilitation in selected individuals. Particularly prominent has been a technique known as constraint induced movement therapy (CIMT), sometimes known as "forced use." In this technique, the unaffected arm is placed in a sling or otherwise immobilized to encourage ("force") the stroke survivor to use the weakened arm. The immobilization is combined with intensive exercises for the weakened arm, for up to six hours each day. The exercises are oriented toward functional tasks, and the patient is expected to keep the immobilizing sling in place and use the weak arm for all tasks throughout the day (such as dressing, feeding oneself, and so on). Treatment programs are intensive but typically last for just two weeks. Several small studies have found that this technique provides some increased use of the arm, even in individuals who sustained their strokes years ago. Moreover, this increase in function appears to be sustained even many months after the completion of the treatment.

This therapy represents an exciting advance for post-stroke rehabilitation but raises many questions as well. How does CIMT work? Will it work for everyone? Can it be used for other parts of the body? Can we get the benefits of CIMT in other ways? The answers to these questions are only partially known, but they are being intensively studied by scientists working in this area. There are several ways in which CIMT might work, but none are yet proven. The originator of the technique, Dr. Edward Taub, initially proposed that part of the reason people do not recover more function in their arms after stroke is that they learn that the arm is not able to perform the needed tasks, and stop trying to use it. At the same time, they learn to function independently without using the affected arm. Despite the fact that the affected arm regains some degree of neurological function after stroke, the stroke survivor is accustomed to managing without its use, and so doesn't integrate recovered abilities into his daily routine. Dr. Taub terms this phenomenon "Learned Disuse." This theory has some appeal but appears to only partially explain the mechanism by which this technique works. We would expect learned disuse to develop over a period of months after a stroke. One study showed, however, that CIMT is helpful even when used within a few weeks of the stroke, an observation that conflicts with the theory of learned disuse (which shouldn't have had time to develop).

Another proposed explanation for the effects of CIMT is that the intensive exercise stimulates the brain to rewire itself to some extent. There are clearly limits to the brain's ability to rewire itself after stroke (known as plasticity), but it is quite possible that this type of exercise program stimulates this ability so that a bit more recovery occurs. We do know from other research that rewiring is part of the process of recovery that normally occurs spontaneously after stroke.

We also know that all people learn new motor tasks and improve them with practice. An example of this is someone who learns how to play tennis and gradually improves his tennis swing. Some people seem to be born with a greater capacity to learn these activities than others, but the fundamental ability to learn a motor task is universal. It seems reasonable to hypothesize that the same ability to learn new motor tasks persists to some extent even after a stroke. A stroke survivor with weakness may never be as adept at a motor task as someone who hasn't had a stroke, but she can still improve somewhat with practice. This type of practice and learning may be part of the mechanism by which CIMT works.

Determining who can benefit from CIMT, and whether it can be extended to other areas of the body, is as important as understanding how the approach works. Because the technique requires a significant degree of pre-existing movement, it is not suitable for individuals with the most severe weakness after stroke. You can imagine the frustration of taking a stroke survivor with no functional use of one arm, tying down her good arm, and asking her to go about her daily activities. This is neither sensible nor effective. The need for a significant level of motor ability to participate in CIMT is a very important practical issue, and one that is not widely appreciated. Another experimental technique, robot-aided rehabilitation, may hold more promise for those with very severe weakness (see below). The question of whether CIMT-type techniques can be applied to other areas of the body, such as the leg, or even adapted to speech problems, is speculative at present. More research needs to be done in this area.

Robot-aided rehabilitation shares certain aspects with CIMT. In this technique, a specially designed robot provides assistance as the stroke survivor attempts certain arm movements directed by the computer. The robot (which looks more like a drill press than it does "R2D2" from *Star Wars*) provides assistance to the patient as he attempt the movements. As the patient improves, the robot gradually provides less assistance. The robot can even be programmed to help with strength training by providing resistance to the movements if the patient is strong enough. Robot-aided exercises are typically provided three to five times per week for four to six weeks.

Robot-aided rehabilitation has been tested in several small studies and, like CIMT, appears to be beneficial both for patients in the early recovery phase and for individuals with long-standing residual weakness after stroke. One significant advantage over CIMT is that the robotic therapy seems suitable even for individuals with very severe weakness in the arm, who would be unable to participate in CIMT. The robot technology is still evolving, and the current units provide exercise only for the shoulder, elbow, and wrist to help the stroke survivor practice reaching movements. This treatment is currently available only in the context of research studies at a few centers (see Appendix p. 246 under "Interactive Motion Technologies"). Robot devices to help retrain walking ability are also being studied (see Appendix p. 245 under "Hocoma AG").

For the legs, a new method known as partial weight-bearing assisted ambulation appears promising. This technique involves suspending the stroke survivor from a harness to reduce the weight he needs to support through his legs while he practices walking after a stroke. The harness is often used in conjunction with a treadmill, and the combination may be more effective than the use of the harness alone. Although this method seems to help some individuals, it is important to recognize that it can't turn a person who is completely unable to walk into an independent ambulator. Rather, it may help someone who is nearly able to walk manage to regain some walking ability, or help other patients who would walk eventually to walk sooner or more efficiently.

CIMT, robot-aided rehabilitation, and partial weight-bearing assisted ambulation are all promising experimental exercise techniques. Because they are experimental and require some specialized equipment, only some rehabilitation centers offer these treatments, and often only in the context of research studies. A full discussion of the pros and cons of participating in clinical research studies is contained in Chapter 20.

Biofeedback

Biofeedback is a technique that has been used for several decades to enhance motor abilities after stroke. Despite multiple research studies on the subject, there is no general agreement on whether biofeedback is beneficial or not. The purpose of biofeedback is to provide the stroke survivor with information about the muscle activity in his weak limb so that he can learn how to control the limb better. For example, someone who is intermittently able to make one of his arm muscles contract slightly after a stroke may have trouble being able to feel if he has succeeded with each attempt. By monitoring the electrical activity in the muscle (using a special recording device on the skin), a biofeedback device provides a visual display (like a light or computer graph) or auditory feedback (a sound that grows louder) showing how much the muscle has contracted. This helps the patient know if he has succeeded and ideally allows him to succeed more easily the next time. Despite its intuitive appeal, biofeedback remains a tool of uncertain utility after stroke. Some centers use it whereas many others do not.

Electrical Stimulation

Another related technique is electrical stimulation of muscles after stroke, sometimes called "functional electrical stimulation," or FES. This technique takes advantage of the fact that electrical stimulation of a muscle will cause it to contract, and the limb to move. Though the theoretical basis remains unclear, some have proposed that FES can help restore normal, spontaneous movements of the affected limb. As with biofeedback, many studies have been conducted but the results are contradictory, and the technique remains controversial.

Biofeedback and electrical stimulation have been combined in a technique called EMG-triggered FES. In this approach, a sensor is placed over the target muscle—for example, the muscle that lifts up the hand at the wrist joint. The patient lifts up his wrist as much as he can. When the sensor detects the muscle contraction, it triggers an electrical stimulation to the same muscle via the same electrode. This causes the target muscle to contract vigorously, "completing" the intended movement (lifting up the wrist). The theory is that by repeatedly performing this cycle, the muscle will become stronger and the control of the muscle will improve. Some research suggests that this does occur, and a commercial unit is available for this type of training (see Appendix p. 246 under "Stroke Recovery Systems, Inc.").

Ataxia

Jane is a forty-seven-year-old woman with a history of hypertension who frequently forgets to take her medications. She develops a cold and uses an old over-the-counter decongestant she has lying around the house. She wakes up the next morning with a severe headache in the back of her head, and she finds that her right side seems to flail around when she tries to move it. She is evaluated in the emergency department, where she is found to have a hemorrhage in the cerebellum, with severely elevated blood pressure. She later finds out that the old over-the-counter cold remedy contained phenylpropylamine (PPA), which the Food and Drug Administration (FDA) removed from the market because of an association with cerebral hemorrhage in women. Jane is told that the damage to her cerebellum has caused ataxia and is responsible for the difficulty she has controlling her right arm and leg. She is puzzled, since the strength in the arm and leg seem good, and she is able to move each of her fingers and bend and extend all her joints. Jane wants to know what ataxia is and why it is significantly affecting her ability to control her right side.

Ataxia is a form of altered motor control with a loss of coordination and/or balance that is very distinct from the weakness and loss of motor control usually seen after stroke. There are two broad forms of ataxia. The most common type of ataxia is known as "cerebellar ataxia" owing to its origins in cerebellar dysfunction. A less common form is known as "sensory ataxia," which results from loss of the ability to feel the location of the limb or trunk in space; this condition results in an uncoordinated movement similar to that seen in cerebellar ataxia.

Cerebellar ataxia can affect the limbs, trunk, or both. If the limbs are involved, movements are often very shaky and tend to become less accurate as the person attempts to reach a target. This can be quite disabling, even though strength and feeling may be normal. Tasks that require precise movement of the limbs, such as feeding oneself, can be quite difficult for people with cerebellar ataxia. Tremors can cause food to spill off a spoon or fork; lack of coordination can cause the individual to hit his face with a spoon as he attempts to reach his mouth. Treatment for limb ataxia often involves the use of weighted implements (for example, a weighted spoon) or wrist weights, which dampen some of the tremors. Exercises are also used, though it is unclear whether they are beneficial.

Sometimes ataxia affects the trunk more than the limbs, resulting in "truncal ataxia." In this condition, the ataxia may not be as evident when the person is at rest or when self-feeding. It becomes most obvious when someone sits or stands, and it becomes clear that she can't keep her body stable in space. Truncal ataxia can severely affect walking because of difficulty keeping the body stable. Walking aids, such as a walker or forearm crutches, may be useful for truncal ataxia, and physical therapy may provide some benefit as well.

12

Loss of Sensation or Vision

Mildred is a seventy-four-year-old woman with a history of poorly controlled hypertension who suddenly develops a severe headache while shopping at the grocery store. The headache is so severe that she sits down in the middle of the store, prompting the manager to call 911. When she is evaluated in the emergency department, she is found to have sustained a left thalamic hemorrhage. She is able to move all four limbs with good strength but seems to have trouble controlling the right side of her body and is unable to walk. Further examination reveals that she can't tell where her arm or leg are located when her eyes are closed. When the physician bends her elbow, she can't report whether it is straight or bent. Even when her eyes are open, she has considerable trouble performing basic tasks with her right arm and leg, despite the fact that she has no weakness. Nor can she feel anything when her arm or leg are touched. She describes them as "numb."

Mildred undergoes extensive rehabilitation but only recovers a small amount of the feeling in her right side. As a result, she is unable to walk and requires a wheelchair. She learns to feed and dress herself with her left arm, because she can't control her right arm well enough to do these tasks. She also develops pain in her right side, which she describes as "like a toothache." She is diagnosed with a central pain syndrome (also known as Dejerine Roussy syndrome). She has no relief with standard pain medications such as acetominophen (Tylenol), ibuprofen (Motrin), or oxycodone (Percocet). She experiences partial relief with gabapentin (Neurontin), however. Why does Mildred have such disability related to sensory loss? What treatments are available?

Loss of Sensation

There are several reasons for Mildred's difficulties. Because there is an intimate relationship between movement and feeling, a person can move in a coordinated fashion only when the brain receives continuous feedback about how the movement is proceeding. Consider the process of picking up an uncooked egg. First, you use your visual system to identify the egg and determine its location. As you reach for the egg, your eyes continue to help guide the reaching task, while at the same time, your sensory system receives information about the location of your hand. If you closed your eyes, you could still probably reach the egg by using this sense of position in your arm. Once you pick up the egg, your sense of touch tells you that you have reached your target. Pressure sensors also tell you how much pressure you are putting on the egg, so that you obtain a firm grip. Without this information, you might not grip the egg firmly enough and drop it, or grip it too firmly and crack the shell.

Performing motor tasks without sensory feedback is analogous to drawing a picture with your eyes closed. You can make the individual movements, but you have no way of knowing if you've made them successfully. Without being aware of the status of your picture, you don't know where to draw the next line, and the resulting picture will be a mess. Similarly, without sensory feedback, any motor task beyond the simplest effort will not succeed.

Sensory loss, or loss of feeling, is quite common after stroke but receives much less attention (and rehabilitation) than loss of movement. Any of the senses can be affected by a stroke. There are more than the so-called five senses taught in elementary school. These include vision, taste, smell, hearing, vestibular (spatial orientation) sensations, and visceral (internal organ) sensations, as well as what is normally thought of as the feeling of touch. Touch is actually a number of interrelated sensations, including fine, discriminative touch (such as the ability to feel the irregularities in the surface of a coin), the more basic feeling of touch (for example, knowing that someone is grasping your arm), pain, temperature, and the very important but often neglected proprioception (knowing where your body part is in space).

Each of these sensory systems can be affected at multiple levels in the brain, with varying results. A loss of fine touch is common with strokes affecting the sensory cortex, but some basic touch sensation is usually preserved even in severe strokes of this area. Strokes affecting the thalamus can lead to complete loss of sensation on one side of the body, which can be very disabling, even if there is no weakness associated with this stroke. Thalamic strokes can also lead to severe pain problems owing to the disruption of the normal sensory pathways in the brain, as discussed in Chapter 17.

Mildred uses visual feedback to help substitute for her loss of bodily sensation. This is generally the most effective compensatory approach for this condition. As with weakness, practicing using the affected limbs is believed to be important in maximizing recovery. There has been very little medical research into rehabilitation techniques for this type of sensory loss, and specific techniques to enhance the recovery of sensation have yet to be developed.

Loss of Vision

Visual information is received by the eyes and then transmitted through the brain to the occipital lobes toward the back of the brain, where it is processed (see Figure 4.1). Because of the way the brain is organized, one half of the visual information from each eye goes to each side of the brain. In other words, the left side of the brain processes visual information coming from the right side of the person. Thus it is common for someone with right-sided weakness to also have loss of vision to the right side after a stroke affecting the left side of the brain. Some people who have difficulty seeing to the right side initially think the problem is with their right eye when in fact the vision to the right side of each eye is affected.

Visual loss of the entire side (left or right) as a result of a stroke is known as a homonymous hemianopsia. If only one-quarter of the visual field is affected (either the upper or the lower half of one side), it is known as a quadrantanopsia. People affected by a quadrantanopsia or even a homonymous hemianopsia may be unaware of or relatively untroubled by their visual loss. This is because we all rely heavily on scanning our environment by looking around and forming a mental "image" of what's around us. As a result, most people can compensate fairly easily and quickly for these difficulties. Initially they may have trouble navigating a busy corridor, reading, or seeing someone to the affected side, but these difficulties tend to improve over time, even if the visual problem persists.

The visual problem can also impact a person's ability to pay attention to the affected side. In these cases, some degree of inattention or neglect accompanies the loss of vision to the affected side. This is often more disabling than the actual loss of vision, since it affects a person's mental "map" of her surroundings. Neglect and attention problems are discussed in further detail in Chapter 13.

Rehabilitation remains limited for visual field loss resulting from stroke. Prism glasses are sometimes used, which essentially shift the intact field of view toward the affected side. These glasses may also be of some use for visual neglect. A new computer-based rehabilitation program developed in Germany appears to provide some benefit in restoring visual field loss after stroke (see Appendix p. 246 under "Novavision"). This therapy should become available in the near future at some centers in the United States.

Double Vision

Double vision, or diplopia, resulting from stroke is a problem not with the eyes but with the parts of the brain that control and coordinate eye movements. Most common after strokes affecting the brainstem, diplopia can be quite distressing and interfere with a broad range of activities. Treatment depends in part on the nature and severity of the eye-movement problem. In cases where one eye has severely impaired movements and control, the best treatment may be using an eye patch to "block out" the visual information from that eye. The brain learns to compensate and ignore the information coming into the patched eye. Patching may also be useful in cases where coordination between the eyes is the major problem. In these cases, the patch may be switched back and forth between the two eyes to give each eye "exercise" while eliminating the double vision. Often with this treatment both eyes will remain unpatched for a period of time in an effort to retrain the brain system controlling eye movements to restore coordinated movements.

In cases in which the eyes are not patched and do not recover coordinated movements, the brain typically "suppresses" the visual information from one eye, so that more normal vision is preserved. Usually the vision is suppressed from the weaker eye, and the stroke survivor relies on the stronger eye for functional vision.

Spatial Orientation

Problems with balance are common after stroke and may result from a number of causes. Weakness and ataxia are both common causes of balance disturbance and are discussed in Chapter 11. In some cases, however, the brain's sense of the position of the body in space is affected by a stroke. When the damage affects the parietal lobe (usually on the right side), a broad range of spatial problems may result, including spatial neglect (see Chapter 13). Some stroke survivors with parietal lobe strokes have an altered sense of midline and have a tendency to fall (and even push the body in some cases) toward the side of the weakness, resulting in instability. Such individuals feel as though they are tilting toward their unaffected side and end up overcompensating by leaning to the weakened side. This condition is known as Contraversive Pushing Syndrome. It can significantly slow down rehabilitation efforts and interfere with mobility and walking. Mirrors are sometimes used to provide additional feedback to the affected stroke survivor, with uncertain efficacy. Many stroke survivors have a gradual improvement in this syndrome over time.

Stroke can also affect balance and spatial orientation by damaging the areas in the brainstem that process information from the vestibular system. This system provides important sensory information on position in space. For example, this sense allows a person with his eyes closed to know whether he is lying flat on his back or standing against a wall. In some strokes affecting the brainstem, this system may be partially damaged, with the result that the stroke survivor may feel as though he is standing on a floor that is tilted. The whole world feels askew, even though the affected person is fully aware of the problem and tries to compensate for it. This condition may be accompanied in some cases by a sense of spinning, known as vertigo. The perception of movement present in vertigo may be associated with severe nausea and vomiting akin to motion sickness. Stroke survivors with vestibular system damage may also develop exaggerated motion sickness, and find that they have difficulty tolerating even short drives in a car. It is important to point out that vertigo has many other causes besides stroke, such as labyrinthitis, which are beyond the scope of this book.

Treatment for loss of balance resulting from a brainstem stroke consists of continued practice with the support of a therapist or family member to prevent falls. Meclizine (Antivert) may be used if vertigo is present, though it is of only partial benefit in most cases. Fortunately, these symptoms tend to improve over time in most individuals.

13

Problems with Memory and Thinking

Harold is a fifty-seven-year-old highly accomplished lawyer who has a history of hypertension, diabetes, and high cholesterol. His career leaves him little time for exercise, eating right, or seeing his physician. While driving to work one morning Harold finds he is unable to control his car. He feels wide awake and is able to speak, but something seems wrong with his vision and he finds the car drifting off the side of the road. Fortunately, he does not injure himself or anyone else when he drives off the left side of the road into a ditch, where he is rescued by the police and emergency medical technician (EMT) squad. The EMT at the scene notes that he has slurred speech and can't move his left side. He is brought to a nearby hospital and is found to have a blocked right carotid artery, and a resulting right hemispheric stroke. He is transferred to a rehabilitation hospital after seven days and is still having difficulty understanding what has happened to him. When I meet Harold, I ask him how his left arm is feeling:

Harold: It feels fine.
Dr. S: I would like to test your left arm strength. Can you lift it up in the air for me?
Harold: OK. (His arm does not move.)
Dr. S: Is it moving?
Harold: Yeah, I think so.
Dr. S: Take a look over here at your arm. Is it moving?
Harold: I'm too tired right now—I'll move it later.

What is going on here? Harold can speak, but he doesn't seem to notice an obvious problem—his left side is paralyzed. Is this condition neurological? Psychological? As we will see, Harold's problems are due to neurological damage to his brain and are a relatively common occurrence after a right hemisphere stroke.

The brain is the location of all thought, motivation, and understanding. A stroke can affect any aspect of these mental processes, and the medical literature is full of examples of how these functions can be damaged by stroke. Certain types of problems and combinations of problems are more common than others, however. Among these are language difficulties, which usually result from damage to the left hemisphere of the brain (see Chapter 15, "Communication Difficulties"). This chapter will discuss some of the other common thinking problems (technically known as "cognitive problems") associated with different types of strokes. Given that the nature of thought is so complex, no discussion of cognition will ever be complete and comprehensive. This discussion will focus broadly on strokes affecting the frontal, parietal, temporal, and occipital lobes and their most common cognitive manifestations.

Right Hemisphere Strokes

Strokes affecting the right hemisphere of the brain can cause a complex set of cognitive difficulties that family members need to understand in order to provide effective rehabilitation and assistance to the stroke survivor. Strokes affecting the comparable part of the left side of the brain (portions of the frontal, parietal, and temporal lobes) typically cause aphasia. Whereas aphasia is usually fairly obvious to a family member, the difficulties seen with strokes affecting the right cerebral hemisphere are often more subtle. Individuals with these types of strokes are usually able to speak and understand but seem to be "off" in their thinking. The most prominent problem affecting people with right hemisphere strokes is usually a striking loss of self-awareness. In the most dramatic cases, the individual is unaware that he has lost any function as a result of his stroke. Like Harold, he may be unaware that his left side is completely paralyzed.

This phenomenon is *not* the same as "denial," which is sometimes seen in someone diagnosed with a severe illness. Denial is a psychological reaction in which the affected person seems to have "forgotten" the diagnosis or the seriousness of the disease. An example of psychological denial would be someone diagnosed with cancer who fails to seek medical attention or treatment because she is unable to accept the reality of her diagnosis. Such individuals remain aware at a subconscious level of their illness but are unable to accept it consciously because it causes too much psychological distress. In contrast, individuals like Harold have "anosognosia," a medical term indicating a lack of awareness of neurological deficits. Harold is truly unable to comprehend that he has suffered a loss of function. While the exact mechanisms of this condition are still debated, it can be conceived of as failure of the portion of the brain that keeps track of the body parts and their functions. With this system malfunctioning, Harold simply can't recognize the problem. Moreover, confronting Harold with the problem just causes him to confabulate, or "make up" an explanation. Confabulation is the damaged brain's attempt to make sense of a situation it doesn't quite comprehend. The confabulation is not an intentional lie, but rather an attempt to fill in the missing pieces of the story. People who are confabulating truly believe they are telling you the truth. Our brains are built to fill in some of the missing details in life—unconsciously we edit the events we observe into a coherent narrative so that we can make sense of our lives. Harold, who is unaware of the fact that his arm is weak, is trying to fit together the pieces of the puzzle he sees by creating a "story" that makes sense (in this case, that he is too tired to move his arm).

Harold is found to have "left neglect," another common problem in people with right hemisphere strokes. Not only doesn't he pay any attention to the left side of his own body; he doesn't pay attention to anything happening on the left side of his world. He looks only to the right side (known as a "right gaze preference") and can't be convinced or tricked into looking to the left. This inability to focus on the left side of the world affects his eating (he only eats the food on the right side of his plate) and even his grooming (he only combs the right side of his hair). When I examine him from the left side, I find that he won't look at me. He hears me but seems to have trouble figuring out where I am. He seems much more interested in the *Jerry Springer* re-run on the TV, even with the sound off, than he does in me. (In truth, I sometimes find this happens with my cognitively intact patients as well, a phenomenon that may be best unexplored.) When I move to his right side (and turn off *Jerry*), he becomes more attentive and is able to conduct a conversation.

After a few visits, he gives me a new answer when I ask him if his left side is weak: "They tell me it's weak. It seems ok to me, but I guess that must be from the stroke." Probing a bit further, I ask him if he can walk. "Sure I can walk, Doc," he replies. When I ask him to get up, however, he has trouble maneuvering with his paralyzed left side and ultimately gives up. Again, he provides a rationalization: "Maybe later Doc—I'm too tired now."

This interchange illustrates another feature of right hemispheric stroke—a lack of ability to draw logical conclusions, even when able to verbally understand the information. For example, a person with this problem may wish to go home prematurely, stating, "I'll be ok at home by myself," even though she knows she is unable to get out of bed without assistance. It is as if each fact is understood in isolation, but the connections between facts are missing. The connection between being unable to walk without help and the ability to go home alone is missing. This difficulty in drawing logical conclusions and recognizing limitations tends to improve over time but may persist in a less obvious form indefinitely.

Harold is severely affected by left neglect. Not only is he unable to pay attention to the left side of his world; he doesn't even recognize that the left side of his body belongs to him. I hold up his arm to show to him, but he doesn't recognize it as his own. This condition is termed "limb agnosia," *agnosia* being Latin for "not knowing." Individuals with limb agnosia may report that their left arm belongs to someone else when asked about it. This lack of awareness poses substantial difficulties for rehabilitation. How can you work on restoring function if you don't even know that the weak limb is your own?

Fortunately Harold, like most individuals with this type of stroke, gradually regains awareness of his left side. Although many techniques have been espoused to restore this awareness, it remains unclear if any of them actually influences the brain's natural ability to recover from this deficit. Gradually Harold comes to recognize first that his left arm is his, and then that the left side of his body is paralyzed. He begins to turn to the left when encouraged, and then eventually turns to the left without encouragement. Despite this improvement, he still tends to be less attentive to events and objects on his left side than on his right. When walking down a crowded corridor, he bumps into objects on the left and needs supervision to walk safely. Guests visit, and he only speaks to the ones sitting on his right. His reading is affected, because he only sees the words on the right side of the page.

How can Harold's family help him when he gets home? Understanding the nature of his difficulties is an important first step. Harold can't be "convinced" to pay attention to his left side. Rather, his family should work with him to reinforce compensatory strategies developed with his rehabilitation team. For example, Harold can use his excellent verbal skills to help him. Some individuals with left neglect work out a verbal "self-reminder" system, whereby they remind themselves to look to the left. When using a cane (as Harold does), he may repeat to himself the order of his walking task: "Cane, left foot, right foot, check left," as he walks down the hall, pausing to look to the left after each step. Other practical actions family members can take include having visitors sit on his right side, removing obstacles (such as a coffee table) from hallways at home, and walking on his left side in busy areas (such as a mall) to protect him from running into unexpected obstacles. Reading may be a particular challenge, owing to his tendency to start reading in the middle of the line rather than at the far-left margin. Some family members place a red mark on the left side and remind the stroke survivor to keep looking to the left until he reaches the line. A strip of Velcro tape can be used in a similar manner; the finger then feels for the Velcro tape as an indicator that the left margin has been reached.

Impulsive Behavior

Some individuals with stroke (especially in the right hemisphere) are "impulsive." Impulsivity is an inability to delay action while considering the consequences. Children are naturally somewhat impulsive and will reach for another's ice cream without hesitation. Some people are naturally more impulsive than others and monitor their own behavior less closely. After a stroke, however, impulsivity may reach a truly abnormal level. A patient with stroke-induced impulsivity may fall repeatedly when getting out of a wheelchair because he can't slow down his intention to get up long enough to lock his wheelchair brakes or reach for his cane. Why some people become impulsive and others do not remains uncertain—some have suggested that baseline personality comes into play.

Frank, who had a stroke similar to Harold's, is very impulsive by nature. His second night in the hospital he falls out of bed, explaining to the nurse who finds him on the floor that he needed to go to the bathroom. Despite multiple reminders from staff, the same thing happens again the next night. Frank explains: "I remember the nurses telling me to call before trying to go to the john, but when I needed to go, I just couldn't wait. I know it was not a smart thing to do, but I just needed to go to the bathroom." Frank is contrite and seems to understand what's going on. Nonetheless, the next night the nurse finds him trying to get out of bed again without assistance. Frank is able to verbalize the appropriate steps he should take to avoid injury, but he can't control himself when the impulse arises. Over time, he is able to verbalize an understanding of his impulsivity but never achieves complete control over it. Why can't Frank control his impulses?

It is tempting to think of the mind as a unitary whole controlled by our consciousness. The mind has many parts, however, and a stroke may affect one part while leaving others intact. This may be hard for a family member to accept, since it is contrary to our own view of ourselves. Often I hear family members complain that their stroke-affected relative "isn't trying." Nothing brings out these misunderstandings more than cognitive deficits. Telling Frank over and over again to wait for help before getting up isn't likely to be very effective, and will lead to frustration for both Frank and his family. A more productive approach may be to build in a delay for Frank—for example, by using a wheelchair seatbelt. Simplifying the environment is another approach. For example, if Frank keeps getting up from a wheelchair without locking the brakes, perhaps he would be safer sitting in a regular (nonrolling) chair rather than a wheelchair when he is resting.

Difficulty Navigating

Professor M. is a seventy-five-year-old retired biochemistry professor who sustains a relatively small stroke in his right parietal lobe. He has some transient weakness that resolves promptly, and he is discharged home directly from the hospital in just a few days. Once he is home, though, his wife notes some peculiar problems. Professor M. has difficulty finding his way around their house. This surprises him, since he feels ok and is able to recall and discuss complex biochemistry material without difficulty. Shortly after returning home, his wife finds him in tears one morning because he wet himself when he couldn't find his way to the bathroom from his kitchen. Gradually he becomes more able to find his way around at home, but on walks in the neighborhood where he and his wife have lived for twenty years, he can't find his own home once it is out of direct sight. Why is Professor M. having such trouble finding his way around, despite the fact that he otherwise seems to have had a good recovery from his stroke?

Professor M. has damage to the portion of his right parietal lobe that is instrumental in forming mental maps of the world and assisting with navigation. People with this type of disability can be highly functional in many regards, but may not be able to leave the house unaccompanied. Recognizing the nature of this problem is critical to preventing affected individuals from getting lost outside their homes. Whereas many people with this problem have other associated damage to the right parietal lobe, some have relatively limited difficulties, which may lead their loved ones to assume that they are fully recovered. As with many cognitive impairments, a key aspect of contending with loss of spatial awareness is recognizing and understanding it. Patients and their families should do all they can to educate themselves about the nature of the problem.

Other Aspects of Right Hemisphere Stroke

Stroke affecting the right hemisphere may cause a number of other cognitive problems. One frequently ignored aspect is loss of the normal rhythm or melody of speech. This condition, known as "aprosody," is due to the loss of the right hemisphere's contribution to normal speech. Speech contains not only words but also important intonations and rhythm, which convey emotion and other meaning. Think of your spouse asking you to perform an undesirable task, such as taking out the garbage. Your response ("Sure, I'd be happy to") can be said in many ways. You might say it enthusiastically, flatly, or perhaps even sarcastically. Although the words are the same, the meaning is different depending on how the words are said. These different meanings come from the prosody of speech. When this is lost, as in aprosody, some aspects of communication are lost as well. Individuals with right hemisphere stroke frequently have a flat, emotionless delivery to their speech. They may also have difficulty recognizing the meaning of others' intonations, and not realize when someone is joking or being sarcastic. Gradual improvement often occurs but may be incomplete. Speech therapy may provide some benefit. It's important for family members to understand what's causing the problem and to be able to distinguish it from depression or lack of interest.

Right hemisphere stroke can also affect social awareness. Individuals with this problem may not recognize or respond appropriately to social cues. They may invade someone's personal space, interrupt people, or not recognize signals that they are embarrassing someone else. This topic is discussed in greater detail in Chapter 14.

Right hemisphere stroke can sometimes impair time awareness, so that the affected individual has difficulty keeping track of the time of day and following the passage of time. The stroke survivor may start asking for dinner before he has eaten breakfast in the morning. He may state that a family member hasn't visited in weeks when that person was actually present the previous day. The person with stroke may have a hard time using a watch or understanding the normal sequence of events ("Which holiday comes after Christmas?"). Timers can help reorient someone to the correct time of day and associated event (for example, taking medication). Calendars and planners are helpful for selected individuals. Motivated individuals sometimes find handheld computers particularly useful.

Other Cognitive Impairments

Memory and Attention Problems

Stroke can affect memory, though usually not to the same extent as other cognitive aspects of brain function. This is partly because both sides of the brain share in forming and storing memories. The temporal lobes are particularly important in memory. One type of injury to the brain that

often causes severe memory damage is anoxic encephalopathy. In this injury (not technically considered a "stroke") certain susceptible structures
in both sides of the brain are damaged due to loss of blood flow and
oxygen supply, including the structures that are involved in forming
memories.

Charlie is a high school science teacher and an avid amateur volleyball
player. His team has had a very good season and is in the middle of an intense playoff game when Charlie suddenly collapses on the ground. His
teammates call for an ambulance, and quickly realize that he is not breathing and has no pulse. They begin cardiopulmonary resuscitation (CPR),
and the ambulance arrives several minutes later. The EMTs find that Charlie has had a cardiac arrest, and they successfully restart his heart using a
defibrillator. Charlie wakes up a few hours later in the hospital but remains
confused for several days. As he becomes more alert, it becomes clear that
his brain has sustained an anoxic injury due to inadequate oxygen supply.
    When Charlie reaches the rehabilitation hospital, his friends and family
are initially quite encouraged. He recognizes them all and seems cheerful
and articulate. He asks about his volleyball team, and when the next game
will be played. All seems well until Charlie states that he is ready to go
home. His friends are a bit surprised, since they were under the impression that he would require several more weeks at the rehabilitation hospital. Just then, his physician walks into the room and warmly greets Charlie.
Charlie responds suspiciously, "Do I know you?"
    His physician responds, "Yes, Charlie, I am Dr. Smith, your physician
here."
    "Well, I don't know you, and I don't think we've met before. Why am I
here anyway?—I feel fine and am ready to go home."
    "As we discussed yesterday, Charlie, you have had a cardiac arrest and
are having some memory problems. You need to stay in the hospital a bit
longer until you are ready to go home."
    "Well, I feel fine, but if you say I need to stay, then I need to stay."
    Charlie's physician leaves, and ten minutes later Charlie is again asking
his friends to take him home. He does not recall the conversation with the
physician; nor, in fact, does he recall any of the conversation he has just
had with his visitors. Why is Charlie able to remember people and events
from the past but unable to learn new information?

Stroke most typically affects short-term memory. This type of memory allows you to recall what you ate for breakfast this morning, or who visited yesterday. By comparison, long-term memory, which is rarely affected by stroke, consists of information and events beyond the immediate past. Examples include remembering your wedding day, or when a child was born. It is important to recognize that short-term memory is also a "holding area" for long-term memories—the first step in being placed into long-term storage. Short-term memory is most severely affected in cases of anoxic encephalopathy, with less severe memory problems resulting from various types of stroke.

Short-term memory problems tend to be most noticeable immediately after a stroke, and then improve over time. Improvement occurs after anoxic encephalopathy as well, though it may be more variable. Occasionally, it will become evident that an older person was actually having significant memory problems *before* a stroke. This may represent the early stages of Alzheimer's disease, which may not have been diagnosed previously, but becomes more obvious when someone is dealing with the physical and emotional stresses of a recent stroke.

A primary strategy for dealing with short-term memory loss is repetition of important information, which often can help overcome a damaged but still partially functioning memory system. Memory aids such as notebooks and planners are frequently used, but people with memory problems often forget to consult these devices. Watch alarms and hand-held computers are particularly helpful for some individuals with persistent short-term memory problems. These tools can help the affected person take medications, keep appointments, and perform other important tasks.

Sometimes difficulties that appear to be related to memory actually reflect another problem altogether: decreased attention. We all know from our school days that you can't remember something that was taught in class if you weren't paying attention. Often it turns out that when a person with a stroke seems to be having trouble with short-term memory, the underlying problem is actually trouble paying attention. Without attention, it is impossible to form new short-term memories.

Attention is a complex phenomenon and involves multiple factors. To pay attention, a person needs to be awake and alert. Someone who is sleepy or drowsy as a result of her stroke will be unable to pay attention.

Even when awake and alert, however, some patients with stroke have difficulty focusing their attention. Attention involves recognizing that something is deserving of attention, focusing attention on that person or activity, and then maintaining that attention in the face of distractions. We all know that we only pay attention to activities that are important to us. This allows us to filter out many of the unimportant stimuli in our environment, such as the humming noise a refrigerator makes during dinner, or the cell phone conversation of the person sitting next to us at the football game. Directing attention to the task at hand requires an ability to recognize the important activity or item requiring attention. Frequently we need to share or divide our attention between two activities. This could involve listening to the radio while driving or, in the case of a stroke patient, negotiating hallway obstacles while correctly placing a cane for walking. Finally, we need to maintain attention. Failure to keep focused on the important task at hand leads to distraction by unimportant stimuli. In the case of Harold, he was unable to maintain his focus on my conversation with him initially, and was instead distracted by the television. Certain stimuli are particularly potent (such as TV, even without *Jerry Springer*). Inability to suppress these distracting stimuli can be hazardous. For example, some stroke patients lose their ability to concentrate on their balance when conducting a conversation. For such a person, a hallway chat can lead to a fall.

Some stroke survivors have difficulty redirecting their attention from one task to the next. They seem to "get stuck" on a single task and may repeat it over and over, despite the clear need to address a new task. This is known as "perseveration." Perseveration can also be seen in speech, when a person keeps repeating the same word or phrase.

From the perspective of family members, the most important approach to helping individuals with attention problems is to reduce distracting auditory and visual stimuli. We all can improve our attention by reducing distractions (I keep reminding my teenage son of this when he's doing his homework in front of the TV), and help keep attention directed where it is needed. The more severe the attention problems, the more important this becomes. Practical examples of reducing distractions include turning off TVs and radios when conversing and avoiding crowded areas such as train terminals during rush hour. Avoid distracting someone who needs to concentrate. For example, do not hold conversations with someone who has attention difficulties while they are walking. Stimulant medications (see below under "Abulia") are often used for attention difficulties, with variable results. Even though they provide only partial improvement, they are often worth trying, since even a small improvement in attention can sometimes lead to significantly greater independence.

Apraxia

John had a stroke three years ago, after which he experienced some temporary weakness of his right arm and difficulty speaking, which rapidly improved. Now he has had a second stroke, this time affecting his left side. He seems fairly alert and aware of his problems but has some unusual difficulties. He recognizes his shirt but tries to put his head through the arm holes. When asked, he can identify the telephone, but he no longer remembers how to dial a phone number. His wife is particularly disturbed to find him one morning trying to comb his hair with his breakfast spoon. When she asks his occupational therapist why he is doing this, the OT explains that John has "apraxia." What is apraxia? Is John confused?

Apraxia has several forms, but they all involve difficulty with complex motor tasks. Someone with apraxia may have good strength and control of the arm (or other body part) but has lost the ability to use it for certain familiar tasks. Common examples include dressing apraxia (as John experiences), tool-using apraxia (John's problems with the spoon and the telephone), and speech apraxia (discussed in Chapter 15). Apraxia can be hard to understand; the affected person appears to have the basic abilities to perform a task but can't put them together. The condition most commonly occurs with damage to the parietal lobes, and is particularly frequent after damage to both sides of the brain in this area. Like most difficulties after stroke, it tends to improve gradually but often incompletely. Some people do fine with "automatic tasks," for example, answering a phone when it rings, but have trouble when asked specifically to perform the same task by a therapist or physician.

Treatments for apraxia are relatively nonspecific, involving practicing small tasks the person finds difficult, and gradually increasing the complexity of these tasks as progress is made. Family members can provide assistance by understanding the nature of the difficulty and allowing extra time for the person to accomplish daily activities. Providing verbal or visual "cues" (essentially reminders and hints) on how to perform a task (say, dressing) is often useful. Family members may find it helpful to sit down with an occupational therapist and review the best way to provide this assistance.

Cortical Blindness

Sara sustains a stroke affecting both of her occipital lobes. It quickly becomes obvious to her family and healthcare team that she has lost her vision as a result. She can no longer count fingers held in front of her, nor find the food on her dinner tray. These functions are usually performed by the occipital lobes, which are responsible for processing visual information obtained through the eyes. Sara's blindness is puzzling, however, in that she doesn't seem aware of it. She states that she can see and tries to go about her activities as though she still can. Since she has no weakness from her stroke, she is able to get up and walk, but quickly trips over a chair and would have fallen if not for an alert nurse. She is willing to accept help but doesn't seem to relate the need for this help to her blindness. How can Sara be blind and not realize it?

Sara is reminiscent in some ways of Harold. Like Harold, she lacks awareness of her stroke-related functional loss. And as with Harold, this phenomenon is neurological rather than psychological. Some individuals with injuries to both of the occipital lobes not only lose vision but also lack awareness of this loss. Isolated unilateral damage (on one side or the other) to the occipital lobes is usually much less disabling and frequently causes a loss of vision to one side (hemianopsia or visual field cut—see Chapter 12), and sometimes an associated visual neglect syndrome (similar to that experienced by Harold). Bilateral damage to the occipital lobes can cause "cortical" blindness (known as "cortical" because damage to the occipital cerebral cortex is the cause), also known as Anton's Syndrome. Like Sara, individuals afflicted with cortical blindness may be unaware that they are blind. As you might imagine, this can be a very disabling condition. Falling and walking into objects are quite common. Compensations used by blind individuals (such as a cane for navigation) are usually ineffective in these people because they don't know they have a problem, and they have difficulty forming a mental "image" of their environment. Individuals with this syndrome may benefit from directly touching objects to locate and identify them. Family members can help by providing spoken information describing objects in the immediate environment.

Recovery from cortical blindness varies and is rarely complete. If severe visual loss persists, stroke survivors often require close supervision by a family member for safety. In some cases, a residential facility (for example, nursing home) is needed to provide this type of supervision.

Lack of Initiative

Sally is a seventy-two-year-old grandmother of three and a pillar of her family. Her daughter works full-time and relies on Sally to care for her fifteen-month-old daughter and four-year-old son. On weekends, Sally often babysits for her son's eight-year-old daughter. Sally's husband of fifty years, Joe, has emphysema from many years of smoking and needs oxygen at home. Although he is able to manage most of his daily activities, Joe relies on Sally for shopping, cooking, and cleaning, and to drive him to his medical appointments. Unfortunately, everything changes for Sally and her family one morning when she sits staring at the breakfast table and complains of a headache. Her husband is puzzled. He asks her to lift up her arms, and she is able to do so, though she responds slowly to him. Joe has read about the warning signs of stroke but isn't sure if this fits. After waiting a while, he calls his daughter at work, and she tells Joe to take Sally to the emergency room. Although the resident who first evaluates Sally doesn't think she has had a stroke, the neurologist who is called in recognizes signs of frontal lobe dysfunction. The head CT scan confirms a large right frontal lobe hemorrhage with mass effect (swelling with pushing on other parts of the brain). Sally is observed closely in the neurological intensive care unit and is stabilized. She is transferred to a rehabilitation hospital after one week, where we meet for the first time.

When I walk in the room, Sally is clearly awake but doesn't seem terribly interested in me. She sits in the bed with a blank expression on her face, and does not respond when I introduce myself. When I ask her name, she replies, "Sally," but then says no more. Nor does she respond when I ask her how she is feeling. "Please raise your right arm," I ask her, but she just looks straight ahead, without moving. When I provide some guidance with my own hand, however, she does raise her arm and seems to have normal strength.

Suddenly the phone rings, and I pick it up and hand it to Sally. She pauses briefly and then says, "The doctor is here now. He's examining me." It becomes apparent that the conversation is over, though she does not hang up nor hand me the phone.

Sally has "abulia"—a lack of initiative. The frontal lobes of the brain are very important in setting goals and knowing when to take action and when to be silent. In Sally's case, the damage has caused her to become "abulic," that is, to lose her initiative. Although she can understand my questions and requests, she doesn't act on them. Using the analogy of a car, it is as if she is stuck in neutral—the engine is running, other systems are working well, but the car doesn't move.

Why does Sally answer the phone when she won't speak to me? While I might be tempted to take this personally, there is no reason to do so. For unclear reasons, the telephone is often a more powerful stimulus than a real live person in the room. Some physicians have even used a telephone call as part of the neurological examination for this condition—a willingness to talk more on the phone than in person helps confirm the diagnosis.

Treatment for abulia is limited. Stimulants, such as Dexedrine (dextro-amphetamine), Ritalin (methylphenidate), Cylert (pemoline), and others are often used, with variable benefits. Modafinil (Provigil) is a new medication that also has stimulating effects and may be helpful in some cases. A few individuals benefit significantly from stimulant medications, but many show modest or no response. Perhaps the damage to the circuitry for this function is too extensive in these individuals to benefit from medication. Fortunately, many people show gradual improvement over time. Sally, for example, improves steadily as the swelling around her hemorrhage gradually subsides. Most individuals like Sally, with damage to only one side of the frontal lobes, have a relatively good prognosis. If both sides of the frontal lobes are damaged, the problem is often more severe and doesn't improve as much over time. This kind of extensive damage is more common with certain types of strokes (bilateral anterior cerebral artery strokes in particular) than others.

Injuries to other portions of the frontal lobe are less commonly due to strokes and can cause problems very different from abulia. For example, damage to other regions can cause loss of normal social inhibitions—almost the opposite of abulia in some sense.

Living with someone with abulia can be puzzling and frustrating. Variable responses are the norm rather than the exception. Sally, for example, becomes more communicative over the course of her recovery and is soon conducting simple conversations with family members. She continues to be "flat" emotionally, not showing the expected range of emotion when her grandchildren come to visit. When asked, she seems to understand what has happened to her but doesn't seem appropriately concerned by it. She returns home with her husband but can no longer be relied upon to care for her grandchildren. She clearly cares about them but cannot be attentive enough to their needs. When asked, she can articulate how she would manage various child-care issues, but her responses seem distant and disengaged. Once she is home with her husband, she tends to sit around the house, showing little interest in her prior activities. Her daughter now shops for her, and a home health aide helps out with the cooking and other household activities. In time her family adapts to her new limitations and establishes a new routine.

In many ways, cognitive effects after stroke can be the most devastating, because they appear to change who a person is. The patterns of behavior, the emotional responses, the judgment and insight that define each person are altered by strokes affecting the portion of the brain responsible for these functions. Family members coping with these life-altering changes need to understand, first and foremost, that these are neurological changes and do not reflect stubbornness or laziness on the part of the stroke survivor. In virtually all cases the person with stroke retains substantial cognitive abilities and should be encouraged to enlist those strengths to help compensate for his losses. Someone with memory loss can still tell or enjoy a joke; a mother with cortical blindness can love and hug her daughter. Family members and healthcare professionals alike must strive to see the abilities, not only the disabilities, of people with cognitive impairments if we are to help them live a rich and rewarding life despite stroke.

14

Emotional and Personality Changes

Bernice is a sixty-three-year-old highly active grandmother who recently retired so she could devote more time to her grandchildren and volunteer for an environmental advocacy organization. Her stroke comes as a complete surprise, and it appears that she will have fairly severe weakness on her right side as a long-term consequence. She remains cheerful and has been asking for extra therapy time while in the rehabilitation hospital. Her rehabilitation team is pleased by her enthusiasm and hard work, but her family is concerned that Bernice doesn't seem to "get it" that she will be physically disabled. Although she clearly knows what has happened to her, she seems excessively optimistic. Her family is worried that she will be devastated when the reality of her condition sinks in. Is their concern justified? Should Bernice be encouraged to face reality?

Denial

Bernice appears to be in denial, a common reaction to a catastrophic event. Denial is common in severe illnesses such as cancer, when a person with a lump may, at some psychological level, "pretend" that the lump is not serious and so fail to seek appropriate medical attention. In Bernice's case, however, the denial is more subtle. Bernice is fully aware of the stroke and its consequences—her denial is of the prognosis. On further questioning, she admits to believing that with intensive therapy and hard work, she will regain full use of her right side.

Denial can easily be confused with anosognosia, a lack of awareness of the effects of the stroke as a result of damage to the brain. This condition is discussed in Chapter 13. Other stroke-related cognitive difficulties can also interfere with a stroke survivor's understanding of his condition, such as problems with memory or focusing attention. In some cases, a mixture of cognitive difficulties and psychological denial is present, and it may be difficult to tease these apart. Family members trying to help someone who doesn't seem to understand the implications or prognosis of his stroke may find neuropsychological evaluation helpful.

Psychological denial is part of a progression of responses to catastrophic illness described by Elisabeth Kübler Ross in the 1960s. The other stages include anger, bargaining, depression, and ultimately acceptance. It is now clear that these stages do not necessarily occur in this order; nor does everyone facing a catastrophic illness necessarily proceed through any or all of them. Nonetheless, this model is helpful for understanding how a person copes with a life-altering event such as stroke.

How should a family deal with denial of prognosis after stroke? The most important concern is whether the denial is interfering with the rehabilitation process. If, as in Bernice's case, the denial is mild and actually enhances the stroke survivor's motivation to get better, then there is no urgent need to "correct" this denial. This does not mean that family members should specifically encourage this response, however. Rather, loved ones should always be open and honest regarding their understanding of prognosis, and make certain that the stroke survivor has access to reliable information from her healthcare team regarding her condition.

Mild denial of prognosis after stroke is common, usually self-limited, and tends not to interfere with the recovery process. Ultimately, the stroke survivor comes to realize that she is not achieving the recovery she expected, despite everyone's best efforts. At the same time, the rehabilitation process has provided her with a set of skills to help her adapt to the remaining disability, and she has begun participating in everyday activities once again. The independence that has been achieved serves as a psychological buffer to the recognition that recovery will be incomplete. This process of moving from denial to acceptance is usually gradual and successful.

In some cases, denial can be more problematic. For example, a stroke survivor may refuse to learn how to dress herself using one-handed techniques, stating, "Why should I learn how to dress myself with one hand?

My other hand is going to be fine." In these situations, the denial needs to be addressed more directly, because it is maladaptive and interferes with the rehabilitation that the patient needs in order to return home. Sometimes, family members or the rehabilitation team can help a stroke survivor through a combination of education and encouragement. If this approach is unsuccessful, family members should seek evaluation by a psychologist or other qualified mental health professional to help the stroke survivor overcome this maladaptive denial.

Bernice returns home and gradually accepts the fact that her right side will not regain normal function. Nonetheless, she remains determined to be actively involved with her grandchildren and she continues her environmental advocacy activities. Her denial has resolved over time and been replaced with an acceptance of her physical limitations and a determination to accomplish her goals in spite of them.

Depression

Phil is an eighty-year-old widower who lives by himself after a stroke that he sustained six months ago. His daughter accompanies him on a visit to his primary care physician, where she expresses concern regarding his loss of interest in his usual activities. Although Phil tells his doctor that he is not depressed, he does acknowledge that he has lost interest in following his local baseball team and no longer feels like joining his long-time friends for their weekly card game. When questioned further, he confides in his physician and daughter that he has been thinking a lot about death. "What's the point of living?" he asks rhetorically. He has been sleeping poorly, waking up at four in the morning unable to return to sleep, and has had a poor appetite recently. Why is Phil so discouraged? Is this a medical problem or just a normal reaction to stroke?

Phil's physician notes that he appears to be depressed, and recommends treatment with an antidepressant. Phil is initially resistant, asking, "How can a medicine fix these problems? Things are just no good, and no pill is going to fix that!" His daughter prevails upon him, however, and he agrees to take an antidepressant. His depression improves; he resumes his card playing and social activities, and he seems interested in his grandchildren again.

Depression is very common after stroke and may affect as many as 40 percent of stroke survivors. We don't understand exactly why stroke survivors so often become depressed, but it seems likely that two major factors contribute to the high risk of depression in this population. The first is the psychological response to a loss of function and the concern that it may not return. Loss of independence frequently leads to feelings of sadness and a grieving for the lifestyle that the stroke survivor previously had and anticipated continuing. Some degree of sadness is common and normal after a stroke and does not require medical treatment. In some more severe cases, however, this sadness develops into a full-blown depression, which can become self-perpetuating and disproportionate to the losses that have occurred.

Second, the actual physical damage to the brain that occurs in a stroke may itself trigger depression. The exact mechanism by which physical damage to the brain causes depression remains unknown. Some scientists have theorized that the loss of brain activity in the area damaged by a stroke affects other areas of the brain, resulting in the development of depression in these other areas. Research attempting to identify specific regions of the brain that could trigger this type of depression after stroke has had inconclusive and conflicting results.

Although it is generally accepted that depression can develop from either one (or both) of these mechanisms, we don't yet know the extent to which these two phenomena contribute to the prevalence of post-stroke depression. Moreover, it is impossible to tell in any given person which one (or both) of these causes is responsible for depression. Fortunately, the issue of how post-stroke depression is triggered remains mostly of theoretical interest, because the same medical treatments work well for most stroke survivors with depression, regardless of the cause.

Identifying a major depression after a stroke can be challenging. Feelings of sadness are very common and may represent a normal reaction to a catastrophic event that results in loss of function. It is hardly surprising that a person who was previously very independent and active would feel sad that he can no longer use his arm or walk without a cane. It may be difficult to discern when this appropriate sadness progresses into excessive sorrow that disrupts a person's ability to move forward with his life. Signs of a developing depression include loss of interest in rehabilitation efforts and therapy, frequent crying, anxiety or irritability, difficulty getting out of bed in the morning, difficulty sleeping, loss of appetite, and loss of pleasure in previously enjoyed activities (for example, spending time with family). Feelings of inappropriate guilt and persistent thoughts of death or suicide can also occur. Whereas some people exhibit very obvious signs of depression, others have more subtle symptoms. Because of their close familiarity with the stroke survivor, family members are often better equipped than anyone else to notice behavioral changes, and should share their observations with the stroke survivor's physician.

Some physicians with limited experience treating stroke survivors may not recognize that depression is present and treatable, and may mistakenly attribute a persistent depressed mood to a "normal" reaction to a disabling stroke. ("Well of course he's depressed—just look at what's happened to him.") Although transient sadness is common and appropriate, more prolonged sadness is often a sign of treatable depression. When there is doubt regarding the need for treatment, a psychiatric consultation is often very helpful in clarifying the diagnosis.

Fortunately, post-stroke depression usually responds well to the same antidepressant medications used for depression in the general population. The selective serotonin reuptake inhibitors (SSRIs), a class of medications that includes Prozac (fluoxetine), Zoloft (sertraline), Paxil (paroxetine), Celexa (citalopram), and others, are frequently effective and usually very well tolerated by stroke patients. Other, newer antidepressants, such as Serzone (nefazodone), Remeron (mirtazapine), and Effexor (venlafaxine), are also usually well tolerated and effective. Some of the older antidepressants, such as Elavil (amitryptiline), though effective, may have excessive side effects and are less well tolerated in general. These older medications are still appropriate in selected circumstances, however, and may be the best choice for a specific individual. Duration of treatment varies widely, with some individuals responding well to a short course of several months of medication, and others requiring long-term treatment. Psychotherapy may be sufficient to treat less severe cases of depression, and it is also an important adjunct in many cases that are treated with medication.

Stroke can be a socially isolating event, and resuming social interactions and outside activities is an important component of treatment for depression. Feelings of loss of value may be prominent in younger individuals who were working before their stroke but are unable to return to their jobs. Volunteer activities that enable stroke survivors to contribute to society are often therapeutic. I have the pleasure of working with a number of my former patients who now volunteer at the hospital where I practice and find satisfaction in helping others undergoing rehabilitation.

Other social supports are available for stroke survivors as well. Stroke support groups exist in many areas (see Appendix) and are often a place where a stroke survivor can feel at ease with other people who have experienced a similar life-altering event. Many support groups are associated with caregiver support groups that may meet separately at the same time. Support groups specifically oriented toward stroke survivors with aphasia exist in some areas to help meet the unique needs of this population.

Maintaining family relationships and friendships is very important as well. Some stroke survivors withdraw from previously important relationships because they feel inadequate or embarrassed. Conversely, friends may feel awkward and be fearful of upsetting a stroke survivor who is visibly disabled. Resuming these social relationships is critically important both for a stroke survivor's successful reintegration into the community and for maintaining a good quality of life.

Religion and other forms of spiritual enrichment are also very important to the recovery process. Resuming attendance at church or synagogue is an affirmation of return to the community. Prayer can provide the spiritual support that many people consider essential as they work through adversity. For some stroke survivors, participating in familiar religious rituals may become more emotionally fulfilling in the aftermath of a life-altering stroke. Some people may even prefer pastoral counseling to services provided by a psychologist or social worker.

Social and religious activities are equally important for caregivers. Caregivers may be tempted to stay at home with the disabled family member rather than continuing to socialize with friends or attend church services. Time spent in these activities may lead to feelings of guilt or abandonment. In reality, however, devoting time to social and religious activities can help sustain a caregiver emotionally and prevent burnout. Maintaining ties outside the home serves the stroke survivor as much as it does the caregiver himself.

Lability

Joyce is a seventy-two-year-old woman who recently left the hospital to live with her daughter after a large stroke affected the right side of her brain. Her daughter is concerned by her mother's ever-changing emotional state. One minute she is pleasant and her usual self, and the next minute she is crying uncontrollably or laughing hysterically. These changes in emotions are triggered by very minor events. Yesterday, Joyce started crying while watching a television commercial that showed a family having a barbecue together. Five minutes later a cell phone company commercial caused her to laugh uncontrollably. Joyce seems aware that her emotional responses are inappropriate, but she can't control them. Her daughter is concerned that she might be depressed, even though her mood seems fine most of the time. What is causing Joyce to have these mood swings? Does she need treatment for them?

Joyce is experiencing emotional lability, a relatively common problem after stroke, though it is often less obvious and severe than in Joyce's case. Lability is a problem of emotional control rather than a mood disorder such as depression. Joyce experiences the same range of emotions as anyone else, but she can't control them as well. Whereas someone without this problem might chuckle at an amusing scene, Joyce can't hold back and laughs uncontrollably. Similarly, she can't control her sad feelings, even if she realizes that a sad commercial on television doesn't warrant tears. Some have termed this emotional lability "emotional incontinence," an apt analogy, since the problem is one of control and keeping emotional expression inside to some extent.

Emotional lability may or may not be associated with depression. In cases where these two conditions occur together, the lability usually manifests as excessive tearfulness, and the excessive laughter noted above may be absent. Depression associated with lability is treated the same as general depression after stroke.

It is important for stroke survivors with lability and their families to understand that the condition tends to stabilize or improve somewhat over time. No specific medical treatment is usually needed, though medications can be used if the symptoms are disturbing to the affected person. Medications used include SSRIs, such as Zoloft (sertraline), Paxil (paroxetine), and others. In Joyce's case, no medication was needed. Both she and her daughter were reassured once they understood the condition and its causes.

Personality Changes

Stroke survivors can experience a broad range of impairments, but personality changes are often the most difficult for family members to accept and manage. Whereas the individual with the stroke may be unaware or only partially aware of personality changes, family members may find them very upsetting, since they strike at the core identity of the stroke survivor. Stroke does not actually create any new personality traits; rather, it takes away certain functions or abilities that served as controls or modifiers of behavior. In a sense, stroke may unmask underlying thoughts or feelings that previously were not expressed or were counterbalanced by other personality traits. Family members often note that their loved ones' mild personality traits became exaggerated after a stroke.

Thomas is a fifty-one-year-old highly educated corporate executive who develops strokes to both frontal lobes as a complication of a brain aneurysm affecting the anterior communicating artery. As a result of his strokes, his personality has changed dramatically. While he retains a broad fund of knowledge and can speak about his work in detail, he now lacks motivation. Previously a highly active individual, he is content to sit and watch television all day. He also has developed odd behaviors whereby he can't help fiddling with things. He will compulsively change channels on the television and play with the remote control continuously if allowed to do so. He picks at his clothing and tears paper cups into many small pieces. His emotional expression is very limited, with a flat, affectless response, even to his children, with whom he was very close prior to his stroke. His children have trouble understanding why their father now seems so disinterested in them and emotionally distant. They find this behavior to be perhaps the single most devastating aspect of his stroke. How can a stroke affect a person's personality so dramatically?

Thomas has some degree of abulia and apathy, which are discussed in Chapter 13. He also has a very limited emotional range and is unable to focus his attention on areas that were once very important to him, such as his family. Personality changes and cognitive limitations often go together, as in his case. Medications can help control some of his behaviors, but they cannot restore his interest and emotional connection to his family. Family members need to recognize this neurological impairment and accept their loved one's limitations to the best of their ability.

Ralph is a sixty-six-year-old recently retired taxi driver who had a large stroke affecting the right side of his brain. He is now living at home with his wife, who says that his behavior has changed and that he is now "uncontrollable." She reports that he does not think about what he says and frequently makes lewd or inappropriate remarks to her, even in the presence of company. He makes crude references to sex, and comments frequently on his wife's weight and physical appearance. She reports that he was previously a fairly quiet man and never spoke in this manner to her. Ralph does not notice any problem, and feels that his wife is too "sensitive" to his "jokes." Has Ralph's personality changed as a result of his stroke? Where did these new behaviors come from?

Ralph is experiencing disinhibition, a phenomenon in which a person does not monitor his behavior as closely as normal. People usually have varying levels of inhibition; some individuals are quite reserved whereas others are very outspoken and share their thoughts freely with those around them. In some stroke survivors, the brain's ability to self-monitor speech and behavior is damaged. In these individuals, thoughts that would have been kept inside are verbalized or acted upon. We all have thoughts that are not appropriate to express or act on in a social setting. Our ability to inhibit these thoughts and actions is an important part of social relationships. For example, it allows a husband to pause and carefully craft an appropriate response when asked by his wife, "How do I look in this bathing suit?" When someone loses this ability, he can say or do things that are not consistent with his personality and values before stroke. Thus Ralph would never have voiced his sexual thoughts in public before, but now he cannot inhibit this speech and makes his wife uncomfortable.

Disinhibition is closely related to impulsivity, discussed in Chapter 13; indeed, many individuals will experience these two problems together.

There is no clearly effective medical treatment for disinhibition, though psychiatric medications are sometimes tried in severe cases. Disinhibition does tend to improve over time, though it may not resolve entirely. As with many other effects of stroke, understanding the causes of this behavior may help family members cope with the problem.

15

Communication Difficulties

Anne is a thirty-nine-year-old woman who sustains a stroke affecting the brainstem. She has severe swallowing and oral motor-control problems, to the point where it is difficult for her to swallow her own saliva. She requires a tracheostomy tube (a tube in the front of the neck for breathing) and a gastrostomy feeding tube for six weeks after her stroke. When the tracheostomy tube is finally removed, her family is discouraged by their difficulty understanding her. It quickly becomes clear that Anne understands everything her family says and is able to formulate sophisticated sentences herself. The problem is that her speech is so severely slurred that it is very difficult for others to understand her. She is having trouble forming the sounds that make up speech, a problem known as "dysarthria." What causes dysarthria? Is there any treatment for it?

Loss of the ability to communicate is one of the most devastating effects of stroke and one of the most misunderstood. Communication disorders can affect the ability to form the sounds of speech (dysarthria) or language itself within the brain (aphasia).

Dysarthria

Dysarthria is due to weakness and loss of motor control of the muscles used to create speech. Although the main voice comes from the vocal cords and larynx in the neck, the tongue, lips, and cheeks all play critical roles in turning this voice into intelligible speech.

In mild cases of dysarthria, family members may find speech easy to understand but slightly slurred. In more severe dysarthria, they may have to pay close attention to understand their loved one. In the most severe cases, the stroke survivor may not be able to generate any intelligible speech. The complete inability to speak owing to loss of muscle control is known as anarthria.

As with weakness of the limbs, dysarthria usually improves over time with speech therapy and specific exercises. Speech exercises include activities to improve the control and strength of the muscles that produce speech. These are called oral motor exercises. In addition, speech compensatory strategies are used to maximize speech intelligibility. One technique known as "overarticulation" is commonly helpful, whereby the person with dysarthria speaks slowly and overemphasizes each sound to provide the listener with the best chance to understand what's being said. Conducting the conversation in a quiet room may also help the listener understand more easily, by eliminating any competing sounds or speech and allowing greater concentration. Familiarity with the speech patterns of the person with dysarthria also helps, and communication may improve over time for this reason, especially with close friends and family. For the majority of people with dysarthria, these approaches are sufficient to allow effective verbal communication.

In a few individuals like Anne, however, the dysarthria is so severe that most people are unable to understand the speech produced. Here technology may be helpful. Some individuals who are able to write using a pencil and pad find this an effective and simple way to communicate. Others, who may have difficulty controlling a pencil effectively, use a letterboard to spell out words. A letterboard is, as it sounds, a board that contains all the letters of the alphabet on it, usually with numbers and a few key words like "yes" and "no." The person uses the board to spell out words by pointing to the letters in sequence. Letterboards are inexpensive and easy to use, but they require the "listener" to be very attentive or risk losing track of the word being spelled out. For individuals with severe dysarthria, computer-based typing devices may be a very helpful alternative to a simple letterboard. These allow a person to type out words, using either a keyboard, if possible, or various switches to select letters. Many of these computer-based systems include speech synthesis, whereby special software "speaks" aloud the typed phrase.

In Anne's case, severe dysarthria is accompanied by difficulty using her limbs, and she is unable to write. She can type slowly, however, and ultimately uses a portable device known as a Lightwriter (see Appendix p. 246 under "ZYGO Industries, Inc.") to type messages to family members that are then spoken aloud by the device.

Changes in the Quality of Speech

In addition to slurred speech, stroke can also result in changes to the sound quality of speech. Weakness of the soft palate can lead to a "nasal" voice, with a higher than normal pitch and altered quality. Speech may sound as though the stroke survivor has pinched his nose closed.

Vocal cord weakness can lead to a soft, breathy-sounding voice that may be difficult to hear. People with vocal cord weakness often find that they can't complete a full sentence without pausing for an extra breath. This is due to the loss of normal breath support. During normal speech, the air in the lungs is slowly exhaled and forms sounds as it passes over the vocal cords. The vocal cords are held together closely by special muscles that form the sounds of speech while also slowing down the exhalation of air from the lungs. When one or both of the vocal cords are weak as a result of a stroke, they cannot be brought together as closely, and the voice produced may be hoarse or breathy-sounding. At the same time, the air escapes the lungs more quickly and runs out sooner, causing the speaker to take another breath mid-sentence.

Aphasia

Ralph is a seventy-two-year-old retired police officer who has a stroke affecting the left middle cerebral artery area. Initially he has some trouble both understanding speech and speaking. Over time, however, his ability to understand speech returns, but he continues to have very limited ability to speak. He can produce some individual words, such as "yes" and "no," fairly accurately, but his speech is slow, halting, and very effortful. A request for turkey for dinner comes out as "Turkey . . . tonight." Ralph seems very aware of his problem and is extremely frustrated by it. How can Ralph understand what is being said but be unable to speak himself? Does he know what he wants to say?

Broca's (Nonfluent) Aphasia

Ralph has a nonfluent aphasia, sometimes known as a Broca's aphasia (named after the neurologist who first described it). He has difficulty formulating and finding the words he needs, though he is able to recognize the correct words when he hears them. Family members may confuse this type of aphasia with dysarthria, since in both cases, the affected person knows what he wants to say but seems unable to say it. In dysarthria, however, the correct words are easily selected by the person but weakness of the lips and tongue prevents him from forming the sounds accurately. In a nonfluent aphasia, the person can formulate the ideas in his mind but can't find the actual words. When the words are found, the person is able to share them with the listener. The experience is analogous in some ways to trying to speak in a foreign language that one has just begun learning. Typically, people with a Broca's aphasia are able to understand what others are saying.

The loss of fluency is another defining characteristic of Broca's aphasia. The speech of someone with a Broca's aphasia has a telegraphic quality and is missing many of the small connector words that form a substantial portion of normal speech. Thus Ralph's request for turkey comes out "Turkey . . . tonight" rather than "Michelle, I would really enjoy turkey for dinner tonight." While the key words are present and the overall meaning can be deciphered, the normal smooth flow (fluency) of words and ideas is missing. This loss of fluency is evident to the stroke survivor and often a source of considerable frustration.

Speech Apraxia

A less common condition is an apraxia of speech. In this situation, the person can formulate the words in his mind but can't properly coordinate the movements to pronounce them. This difficulty in forming the sounds is disproportionate to the apparent weakness of the muscles, which may be otherwise strong and functioning well. People with speech apraxia often report that even speaking simple words feels like speaking a complicated tongue twister. We can think of apraxia as a sort of high-level motor coordination problem, and dysarthria as more of a basic weakness problem. To complicate matters further, apraxia can occur in conjunction with a Broca's aphasia, and it may be hard to determine how much of the verbal fluency problem consists of finding the words (aphasia) versus forming the sounds (apraxia).

Speech therapy is important for the treatment of nonfluent aphasia and apraxia. Practicing speaking in a supportive environment appears beneficial, and family members can play an important role by providing opportunities for this practice. Speech therapists have employed a variety of treatment approaches, such as melodic intonation (trying to "sing" speech to take advantage of the unaffected side of the brain), though no single approach has been found to be the most effective.

Anomia

Another common speech problem is difficulty finding individual words, known as "anomia." This inability to find specific words, though sometimes present in other aphasia syndromes such as Broca's aphasis, is the cardinal feature of an anomic aphasia. In people with anomia, speech flows normally (in sharp contrast to Broca's aphasia, where loss of fluency is a key feature), but individual words cannot be retrieved when needed. Many people with anomia compensate by using substitute words that are close in meaning, though incorrect word substitutions (paraphasic errors) can occur. Working around a missing word by using a phrase to substitute is known as circumlocution, and is also common. An example of circumlocution is "the place where they sell things" instead of "store." Circumlocution can also be used as a therapeutic strategy—as a way to make one's intent known, even when the specific word can't be recalled.

Sadie has a form of aphasia known variously as a nonfluent aphasia, Wernicke's aphasia, or receptive aphasia. In some ways, this condition is the inverse of a Broca's aphasia. Sadie can speak fluently but doesn't understand speech. This can be a particularly severe communication disorder, with confusion and agitation often resulting. Sadie speaks non-stop but doesn't make any sense. Moreover, she makes up new words that seem to be constructed of parts of normal words. For example, she greets her daughter with the sentence, "Salad so happy you brought the sixmaker. Can we go footblue now? I want to go footblue!" As you can imagine, her daughter doesn't know what to make of this utterance. It's clear that Sadie is trying to communicate an idea but it's impossible to know what this idea is. Attempts by her daughter to have her clarify her meaning just compound the problem. Sadie, like many individuals with this type of aphasia, seems unaware that she has a problem. She gets angry at visitors when she can't understand their speech, or if they fail to respond to her own attempts at communication.

As with other aphasias, a Wernicke's aphasia often improves over time, though to a variable extent. In less severe cases, communication is reestablished, but frequent word substitutions may persist, and made-up words are included in speech. A persistent severe Wernicke's aphasia is severely disabling.

Mixed Aphasias

Lee is a seventy-two-year-old woman whose stroke causes a fairly severe loss of speaking ability, though she is alert and attentive and tries to communicate. Her family is puzzled by the discrepancy between what she seems to understand and what her speech therapist is reporting to them. When they spend time with her, she pays close attention and nods appropriately. She seems to recognize all her close family members, and to understand everything that is happening around her. Lee's speech therapist reports, however, that Lee is having trouble understanding any speech except the most simple statements. Why does Lee seem so much more impaired to the speech therapist than to her family?

Lee has a mixed aphasia, with a combination of comprehension and language-fluency difficulties. As in Lee's case, it is common for an aphasic stroke survivor to have mild to moderate difficulty with speech comprehension accompanying a more severe language-fluency deficit. It is often difficult for family members to get an accurate sense of someone's ability when they are unable to have a back-and-forth conversation. Often the stroke survivor's ability to understand seems better than it truly is. This is because the person with aphasia is trying very hard to connect socially and emotionally with her family member. It is common for people with aphasia to nod as if agreeing or understanding, but to have missed the actual meaning of the conversation. Medical professionals who are not experienced with aphasia may make similar (and understandable) mistakes, and assume that someone understands more than she is able to, on the basis of these same nonverbal interactions. Rehabilitation professionals often test comprehension by asking someone with aphasia to perform a simple task, such as picking up an object out of a group of objects, or pointing to someone in the room. These simple requests provide insight into how much information is actually registered by the person with aphasia.

Many people with mixed aphasia experience significant improvement in comprehension over time, even if they are left with substantial difficulties expressing themselves verbally. Improvement in language fluency and language comprehension may not occur at the same rate or to the same extent. Family members should recognize that limited progress in verbal expression doesn't mean that comprehension isn't improving more rapidly.

Global Aphasia

Burt is a sixty-four-year-old man who developed a blocked left carotid artery owing to hypertension, diabetes, and high cholesterol. As a result, he has lost all ability to communicate verbally, and his family is told that he has a "global aphasia" (also known as "total aphasia"). Burt's aphasia involves both comprehension and the ability to speak, and is the most severe type of aphasia. Does Burt understand what is happening? Is any communication possible?

Although global aphasia indicates a loss of both the ability to speak and the ability to understand speech, there are nonetheless important gradations of severity within global aphasia, and often substantial ability to communicate is still present. Some people with this condition are able to comprehend basic gestural communication. True sign language, such as American Sign Language (ASL), is affected by aphasia the same way that speech is, since aphasia is a disorder of language processing, not the mechanics of speech production, and ASL is simply another form of language. At a more basic level, however, the ability to understand simple gestures such as "come here," "stop," or pointing to the object of interest using common gestures is often better preserved than the ability to create or understand spoken speech. Some family members find it helpful to use gentle guiding touch to indicate the desired idea (for example, "turn this way"). The ability to understand these "tactile" forms of communication is commonly preserved even in severe aphasias. In addition, creating an environment or situation that makes the desired activity evident visually—for example, by setting out food to encourage someone to eat and then handing him a fork—can be an effective means of nonverbal communication.

Other compensatory techniques include the use of communication boards with pictures or photographs of key objects and people, for example, close family members, food, the bathroom, and so on. While some patients and families find these very helpful, many feel that other nonverbal communication techniques, such as pointing and gesturing, are more effective.

Automatic Speech

Many people with aphasia find that they can produce some words unexpectedly and clearly. These are typically exclamations or short, frequently used phrases such as "Oops," "Hi," or "See you later." These words and phrases are often called "automatic speech," because the brain seems to produce them without the usual process of formulating a thought and then speaking it aloud. These phrases are uttered without thinking. Many people with aphasia have some preservation of this type of speech. Unfortunately, by its very nature, automatic speech can't be used intentionally, and the same words may be difficult or impossible for a person to speak deliberately. Cursing is a very common form of automatic speech, and some people with aphasia find themselves cursing more than they did before their stroke.

Perseveration

Some people with aphasia find that they get "stuck" on a word and keep repeating it, even when inappropriate. For example, when shown a book, the aphasic individual may be able to identify it accurately. Then, when shown a key, the person may again identify it as a book. This is known as perseveration. When caused by aphasia, perseveration is generally not a failure to recognize the object and its appropriate use but rather a type of word substitution. Perseveration can also be seen in people who do not have aphasia, but have other types of cognitive dysfunction—in these individuals it represents an inability to switch from one idea to the next rather than a language disturbance.

Non-Native English Speakers

Aphasic people for whom English is a second language may find it easier to communicate in their native language. It is rare for someone to completely lose the ability to speak one language and retain the ability to speak another, but the most familiar language is usually the best preserved. Decisions regarding the language used for speech therapy need to take into account the language the stroke survivor will need on a daily basis. Do family members and friends speak his native tongue? Other practical issues include the challenge of locating a speech therapist fluent in the stroke survivor's native language or providing therapy via a translator. For these reasons, speech therapy is often provided in English, even if the native language is somewhat better preserved.

Can People with Aphasia Think?

Family members often wonder how someone with aphasia after a stroke thinks. Our conception of thinking generally includes an internal verbal commentary, and so it seems logical that problems with language would result in problems with thinking. In fact, however, much of our daily thought does not involve language directly. For example, consider the thinking process of a person crossing the street. The first decision to cross the street is a conscious one, but one that does not generally include thinking the words, "I'm going to cross the street now." Moreover, when a car is observed coming toward the intersection, the decision to wait for the car to pass similarly does not involve any internal "speech." In fact, it is easy to devote the brain's language abilities to an unrelated activity while crossing the street, such as chatting with a fellow pedestrian. This example illustrates that much of our daily thought is independent of language. As a result, these aspects of thinking are less affected by aphasia.

For someone with aphasia, much of the daily thinking that does not involve language continues unimpeded. Thus a person with aphasia can decide which of the foods on her plate she wishes to eat, which blouse to wear, and whether a visitor pleases her or is unwanted. Many of the more abstract thought processes, however, do seem to rely more heavily on internal language. Politics, religion, and even planning next summer's vacation are all more abstract than deciding what to eat, and thus more severely affected by aphasia. For people whose aphasia is predominantly nonfluent, many of these internal thoughts continue but may be very difficult to communicate. Abstract conversations about the meaning of life are typically much more problematic than more concrete discussions about where to go for dinner, or which family member should host Thanksgiving this year.

From a family member's perspective, the extent of the impact of aphasia on the stroke survivor's thinking abilities will take time to understand fully. The important thing is to make no assumptions in either direction: Don't assume that someone's thought processes are normal, and don't presuppose any specific limitations. Give the person a chance to demonstrate his abilities, so that he can participate in running his own life as much as possible.

All people with aphasia benefit from patience and understanding on the part of those communicating with them, which may be challenging and time-consuming. Allowing sufficient time for communication, communicating in a quiet and nondistracting environment, and continuing social interaction are all helpful strategies to cope with this disorder. Support groups are often helpful for individuals with aphasia, who may share strategies and socialize in a supportive environment. The National Aphasia Association (see Appendix) is devoted to aphasic people and their families. The association works on advocacy issues for individuals with aphasia and also provides information on local aphasia support groups.

Reading and Writing

Reading and writing are important skills that are often affected by aphasia. Since aphasia is a disorder of language, not of speaking, it follows that problems with speech and verbal comprehension are accompanied by similar problems in reading and writing. Most aphasic individuals communicate best by speaking and listening, but a significant number actually find it easier to read and/or write. Writing is a skill that requires considerable control of the hand and arm muscles, however, and so the hand weakness that sometimes accompanies stroke can be as much of an impediment as aphasia. Speech therapists include work on reading and writing as part of their therapy program, and occupational therapists may also work on writing, since it involves fine motor skills of the hand. Aphasia can also affect the ability to manage numbers and mathematics, thus making tasks such as writing checks challenging.

The degree of recovery varies and may be less complete than the recovery seen in speech and speech comprehension. The person with aphasia often needs assistance with practical tasks involving reading and writing. The support of family members and friends can be enormously beneficial in helping the person adjust to new limitations.

Aphasia and Independence

Tony sustains a stroke that results in severe nonfluent aphasia. He has good language comprehension and communicates reasonably effectively with his wife and a few close friends. His physical abilities were not affected by the stroke, and he has always enjoyed walking. He has made it clear to his wife that he would like to walk around the city by himself. His wife is very concerned about this possibility, fearing that he will get lost or injured: "What if he gets sick—how will he let them know what's wrong with him? How can he contact me if he needs help?"

Can a person with aphasia go out into the community alone? Can he live by himself? In many cases, the answer to these questions is yes. With some simple preparations and precautions, a person with aphasia can live an independent life without much regular assistance from anyone else. In order to do so, however, the person must have fairly good ability to understand spoken language. Although individuals with global aphasia generally require twenty-four-hour supervision, those with severe nonfluent aphasia can often achieve high levels of independence. Rehabilitation specialists can provide guidance regarding the amount of supervision a person needs, though it is important to recognize that these recommendations will be somewhat subjective, and the need for supervision frequently changes over time.

A person with severe aphasia should take certain precautions to remain safe in the community. He should carry a list of contact information for emergencies and a brief written explanation of his medical problem in case of emergency. Some people find emergency alert systems reassuring. In case of an emergency, they simply press a button and local emergency response providers are notified. These systems are often helpful for stroke survivors with aphasia who are living alone or spending time alone in a home setting. A cell phone may be useful in some situations, though the ability to use it effectively varies with the type and severity of the aphasia and/or apraxia. Some people with aphasia like to have a family member present for physician visits, as a means of sharing information with the family member, and also to help ask questions on their behalf, though others do not find this necessary or desirable. In the latter case it's often helpful to provide the physician's office with a telephone number of a non-aphasic family member in case the office needs to contact the patient by phone to share a laboratory result or reschedule an appointment.

For many people, being able to function independently is a cherished ability and one that they will not (and should not) give up easily. Understanding these issues and working with the aphasic stroke survivor to reestablish this independence is an important goal for family members.

Depression and Aphasia

Depression and other mood disturbances can complicate aphasia. The diagnosis and treatment of depression are more difficult in people with aphasia because medical personnel rely heavily on verbal communication to assess mood and other symptoms. Nonverbal signs and symptoms of depression can often provide substantial information, however, and family members should be sure to report them to the stroke survivor's physician. These nonverbal signs include frequent tearfulness, pushing away or turning away from close family members, loss of initiative, loss of interest in getting out of bed, and sleep and appetite disturbances. Whereas traditional psychotherapy may be difficult in cases of aphasia, antidepressant medications appear to work as well for these individuals as for anyone else with depression. The key is to recognize depressive symptoms and seek treatment for them.

Singing

Singing is largely a function of the right side of the brain and is often spared in individuals with left hemisphere strokes resulting in aphasia. This dissociation between speech and singing is the basis for a type of aphasia therapy known as melodic intonation in which speech is "sung" instead of spoken. This technique is of variable therapeutic value, though selected individuals may find it useful. Some individuals with aphasia find that singing allows them to express themselves vocally when speech is difficult. I have had the pleasure of hearing a stroke survivor with aphasia deliver a technically impressive and enjoyable singing performance, even though she has difficulty conducting a conversation. Singing can thus be a valuable form of vocal self-expression for someone whose verbal abilities are otherwise limited.

Early after a stroke, family members should have a careful discussion with the physician and speech therapist to understand the nature and extent of their family member's speech and language difficulties. Loved ones should strive to avoid overestimating or underestimating the ability of the patient to participate in medical or personal decisions. Even if someone is severely affected by a stroke, it is important to recognize improvement as it occurs, so that someone who is able to participate in his own life decisions is not unnecessarily excluded from this process. At any stage of recovery and with any severity of aphasia, family members should work to maximize effective communication with the stroke survivor and ensure his involvement in important decisions regarding his medical care and other aspects of life.

16

Swallowing Difficulties

Mike is a sixty-two-year-old house painter who suddenly becomes dizzy while working. He also reports trouble swallowing and severe coughing. Mike is diagnosed with a stroke affecting the brainstem and is admitted to the hospital. Because of his severe swallowing difficulties, a tube is threaded through his nose down into his stomach (known as a nasogastric tube, or NG tube). He is fed through this NG tube, and no food or drink is given by mouth. Over the next few days he continues to be unable to eat, and the decision is made to place a tube directly into his stomach (known as a gastrostomy tube, or G-tube). He then spends a few weeks at a rehabilitation hospital and resumes walking and managing most of his daily activities. His swallowing remains quite limited, however, and he returns home with his gastrostomy tube in place. He and his family are quite anxious about this tube, though they successfully learn how to use and care for it. A few months later his swallowing has improved sufficiently to remove the tube, though he still needs to eat slowly and use certain techniques the speech therapist taught him to keep his swallowing safe. Why did Mike have so much difficulty swallowing? Will he eventually recover completely?

Difficulty swallowing, also known as "dysphagia," is a common symptom of stroke and can lead to nutritional problems, medical complications, and disruption of a person's lifestyle. Although the majority of people with dysphagia improve considerably, some have lifelong problems, and a few may be completely unable to resume eating. Eating and swallowing depend on multiple brain functions, including the ability to bring the food to the mouth, stay focused on the task of eating, feel the food in

the mouth and throat, have sufficient muscle strength to chew and ma-
nipulate the food in the mouth, and have the coordination to make certain the food moves at the right time and place. Stroke can affect any or
all of these functions.

Strokes affecting many areas of the brain can cause dysphagia. Any
stroke that causes weakness of the arm and leg can also cause weakness
of the swallowing muscles. Stroke affecting the brainstem, as in Mike's
case, may cause particularly severe dysphagia. Strokes affecting the motor and sensory parts of the brain (for example, the frontal and parietal
lobes) can cause dysphagia as well.

The Swallowing Process

Eating is a complex activity with several stages, each of which can be a
source of difficulty. The first stage of eating is obtaining and preparing food, then bringing it to the mouth. Stroke patients who have a variety of cognitive difficulties may find this to be the limiting factor in their
eating. An example would be someone who is having trouble staying
alert and focusing attention shortly after a stroke (see Chapter 13). Although the swallowing function might be reasonably well preserved, eating while not alert can lead to choking. Alternatively, if a stroke survivor
has problems with attention, he may have trouble staying focused on his
meal, or forget that he is in the middle of chewing food. If he has apraxia
(see Chapter 13), he may have trouble using his utensils correctly. Some
individuals are impulsive after a stroke and have trouble pacing themselves through a meal. They may stuff their mouths with food faster than
they can chew and swallow it, leading to a risk of choking.

Once food has been obtained and brought to the mouth, the swallowing process begins with the "oral phase."

Oral Phase

The first phase of swallowing, the oral phase, involves taking the food
into the mouth, chewing it, forming it into a moist lump, and moving
the lump of chewed food from the front of the mouth to the back of the
mouth. Individuals with attention problems (particularly left neglect) or
those with sensory loss on one side may tend to "pocket" food in the

cheek inadvertently. Since they are unaware of this food, it presents a hazard; it can dislodge unexpectedly and cause "aspiration" (when food goes "down the wrong pipe" toward the lungs rather than the stomach). Foods that are very soft, such as purees and puddings, are less prone to pocketing and are easier to move from the front of the mouth to the back. For this reason, these foods may be the safest options for someone with this type of dysphagia.

Spillage out of the side of the mouth can be a problem for someone with weakness and/or sensory loss on one side of the mouth. In this situation, the individual may drool or dribble food out of the weak side.

Sensory loss can also affect chewing. If sensory loss is severe, the stroke survivor may have a tendency to bite her tongue or cheek. With practice, most people can learn to compensate for this problem over time.

Normally, when food has been chewed, it is formed into a soft lump by the tongue known as a "bolus." The bolus is then pushed by the tongue to the back of the throat. When the tongue is weak as a result of a stroke, there may be difficulty in forming and controlling the bolus. Foods may slip past the tongue prematurely. This is known as "premature spillage," and it can cause the food to go down into the throat before the throat is prepared. This can result in aspiration. Liquids are particularly difficult to control, and "thin" liquids (such as water) are the most difficult. At the other extreme, dry, crumbly foods, such as crackers, need to be carefully chewed and mixed with saliva before they are propelled backward in the throat. If not, a small dry crumb can tumble backward prematurely, leading to aspiration.

Normally, when the food bolus is brought to the back of the mouth (also known as the "pharynx"), it initiates a reflex action in the pharynx to swallow the food. This next stage is known as the "pharyngeal phase."

Pharyngeal Phase

The second, pharyngeal phase of the swallowing process is what we usually think of when we speak of "swallowing." This stage of swallowing can be initiated voluntarily (in other words, you can swallow when you choose to), but once it is started, it is automatic and not under a person's conscious control. It is largely automatic during normal swallowing—once the food bolus is pushed back, the pharyngeal swallow is triggered without conscious thought.

The pharyngeal phase of swallowing is complex and involves multiple coordinated activities to bring the food into the esophagus (the tube that connects the throat to the stomach) while simultaneously protecting against food entering the lungs. In normal swallowing, the tongue pushes the food bolus back toward the upper end of the esophagus, while the larynx (commonly known as the "voice box," or "Adam's apple") is pulled forward under the base of the tongue (and out of the way of the food bolus). The muscles in the pharynx then constrict in sequence to help push the food down toward the esophagus. At the same time, a structure known as the epiglottis (see Figure 16.1) automatically tilts down to protect the entrance to the larynx. If this structure fails to function properly (as can occur with stroke), food may go down into the larynx and head toward the lungs (see "Aspiration" below). Finally, the opening to the upper end of the esophagus, known as the upper esophageal sphincter, relaxes and allows the food bolus to enter into the esophagus. When the swallowing system functions properly, the food is then transferred from the pharynx to the esophagus.

Esophageal Phase

Once the food has passed through the pharyngeal stage, it heads into the third phase, when it enters the esophagus, a tube connecting the end of the pharynx to the stomach. Stroke doesn't usually directly affect esophageal function very much, so this phase is rarely a problem after stroke. Other medical disorders can, however, affect the esophageal phase of swallowing. These conditions will often cause a sensation of food being "stuck" in the chest, or of pain when the food passes through the chest. Unlike stroke-related dysphagia, these esophageal problems are usually least severe with thin liquids, providing another way to distinguish the two types of problems. If these symptoms are present, it is an indication that another, unrelated swallowing problem may be to blame. Different types of tests may be needed to evaluate these symptoms, which are beyond the scope of this book.

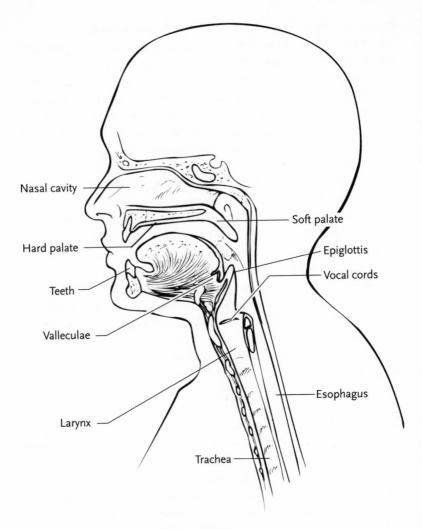

FIGURE 16.1   *Diagram of swallowing structures.*

Aspiration: When Swallowing Goes Awry

The underlying risk for people with dysphagia is of aspiration, or of having food or liquids go into the lungs instead of the stomach. Everyone aspirates small amounts on occasion, and usually responds with vigorous coughing to clear out the breathing passageways. In dysphagia, however, the frequency and amount are greater than usual, as are the risks. Aspiration can result in episodes of "choking"—in truth, coughing fits caused by food or liquids going down the breathing passageways rather than into the stomach. If enough material is aspirated, it can actually block off the breathing passageways entirely—a medical emergency. Lesser amounts of aspiration can lead to pneumonia, the most common concern in dysphagia. Occasionally, individuals who chronically aspirate small amounts of oral contents may avoid pneumonia but may gradually develop long-term damage to the lungs over many years.

The body has several "back-up" lines of defense in case aspiration occurs. The first defense is the larynx. The vocal cords, in addition to forming the sounds of speech, normally close during swallowing to prevent the entry of food down further past the larynx into the trachea (the tube that leads to the lungs). Unfortunately, the vocal cords may be weakened by stroke, and this defense system may be malfunctioning as well.

If food does slip past the vocal cords, the next line of defense is the cough reflex. While many think of cough only as an annoyance that results from a pulmonary infection, it is actually a very powerful protection for the lungs against foreign materials. When food or another foreign substance lands in the tubes leading to the lungs (trachea and the bronchial tree), it irritates them, triggering a cough reflex. This reflex is designed to push air out very forcefully and quickly, and, ideally, carry out the undesirable substance with it.

Coughing is the body's major defense in cases of aspiration. Some individuals have a damaged coughing reflex and do not cough, choke, or even realize when they aspirate. This "silent aspiration" may be more hazardous than the more obvious aspiration, even though it causes fewer immediate symptoms. When someone has silent aspiration, he fails to cough out the foreign material, which can then lodge in the lungs and cause pneumonia to develop. In contrast, someone who has a strong cough reflex is usually able to cough vigorously and clear the dangerous material out of the breathing passageways.

People with dysphagia can aspirate even without eating. Saliva is produced continuously in the mouth and needs to be swallowed to avoid drooling or accumulation in the back of the throat. Individuals with severe dysphagia may be unable to swallow their own saliva, and so they end up aspirating it. Saliva is full of bacteria, and aspirating it can thus lead to pneumonia.

The final level of defense is the body's immune system. The immune system relies on special infection-fighting cells known as white blood cells and related cells to attack infections. Saliva or food that does reach the lungs contains many bacteria from the mouth. The lungs contain white blood cells and can usually successfully fight off an infection in cases where only a small amount of food reaches the lungs. If too large an amount reaches the lungs, however, a full-blown pneumonia can get started, requiring antibiotics for proper treatment.

Assessment of Dysphagia

Several techniques are used to determine the safety of swallowing, and to identify the most effective means of treatment and/or compensation for dysphagia. The first of these techniques is a careful clinical assessment by a speech therapist. This includes examination of the muscle strength, control and coordination, sensation, vocal quality, and the ability to swallow in a timely fashion. Depending on the severity of the dysphagia, small amounts of food may be provided to test the ability to swallow different consistencies (for example, thin and thick liquids, pureed foods, and so on).

In some cases, clinical assessments of swallowing are inconclusive, and further diagnostic tests are needed. The most commonly used test is an x-ray study of swallowing, known as a videoflouroscopic swallowing study (also known as a modified barium swallow). This test records an x-ray "movie" of swallowing. Liquids or foods containing a substance visible on the x-ray (barium) are given so that the ability to swallow these substances can be recorded. Certain compensatory maneuvers (see below) may also be tried during the test to determine their efficacy in preventing aspiration. These x-ray studies are generally performed by a speech therapist in conjunction with a physician. This test takes five to fifteen minutes to complete in most cases.

In some institutions, a different technique is used to provide information about swallowing ability. This technique is known as a fiberoptic endoscopic evaluation of swallowing (FEES). It involves placement of a small flexible viewing device (endoscope) through the nose into the back of the throat. The structures responsible for swallowing are examined, and portions of the swallowing process are observed through the endo-scope. This technique provides less complete information about swal-lowing than a videoflouroscopic swallowing study, but it may be more readily available in some institutions.

Another technique involves the use of a blue food-coloring dye. This technique is most commonly used for people who have a tracheostomy tube. The test involves placing a small amount of blue dye in the patient's mouth or in food. The presence of blue dye in the phlegm coughed or suctioned out of the tracheostomy tube indicates that some portion of the blue dye has been aspirated. The usefulness of this technique remains controversial, since the presence of blue dye in the suctioned or coughed material may not accurately predict pulmonary complications (for exam-ple, pneumonia).

Managing Dysphagia

In some cases, the swallowing evaluation will indicate that someone is at high risk of aspiration and should not be fed orally at the present time. In these situations, a feeding tube is typically used to provide nutrition, fluids, and medication until swallowing improves sufficiently to resume eating safely. In other cases, the problems are less severe and can be managed with the use of a modified diet and/or special swallowing tech-niques.

Mild dysphagia can be managed by modifying the diet and taking safety precautions without the need for extensive swallowing therapy. In such cases, a soft diet and eating slowly may be sufficient for someone to resume eating immediately after a stroke. Speech therapy is helpful to provide training in compensatory techniques and strategies, as well as to perform periodic reassessment of swallowing abilities.

For cases of intermediate severity, the use of special diets and/or phys-ical maneuvers to improve the safety of swallowing can allow someone to eat safely again. In these cases supervision and intensive therapy by a speech therapist are required.

Swallowing Techniques

Several techniques have been designed to help people with dyspha-gia swallow as safely as possible. Bending the head forward, commonly known as a "chin tuck," is often helpful in reducing aspiration. This simple maneuver provides significant benefit in many individuals. Depending on the specific nature of the swallowing difficulty, other maneuvers, such as turning or tilting the head to one side or the other, may be useful. Some individuals are helped by a "double swallow," whereby they make certain that everything in their mouth and throat has been successfully swallowed by repeating the swallow twice for each bite. The speech therapist works with the stroke survivor to determine which strategies will be most effective in minimizing the risk of aspiration.

Coping with Special Diets

As discussed above, certain consistencies are easier to swallow than others, with thin liquids (like water) and crumbly dry foods (like crackers) being the hardest items for someone with dysphagia after a stroke. Often individuals return home after a stroke still requiring a special diet, which can present a significant challenge for their families. This challenge is particularly difficult when trying to prepare appealing and tasty meals within these dietary restrictions. A cookbook for people living with dysphagia, the *Non-Chew Cookbook,* is available (see Appendix).

As a rule, any food can be ground or pureed to the point that it can be eaten by a person with dysphagia. Some foods, like soup, lend themselves very well to pureeing, and a hearty, thick soup may be more appealing than a shapeless lump of puree on a plate. Home-prepared foods tend to be more palatable but more labor-intensive to prepare than commercially available foods (for example, baby foods, yogurt, applesauce). Thickened liquids are commonly required by people with post-stroke dysphagia. Liquids can be thickened to various degrees, depending on the severity of the dysphagia. Thickener powder (Thick-it and others), which consists of cornstarch, can be used at home. A mildly thickened liquid is often referred to as having a "nectar" consistency. Generally, one tablespoon of thickener powder added to four ounces of liquid will produce a "nectar" consistency. More heavily thickened liquids are often referred to as having a "honey" consistency (this term is a bit confusing, since honey is very syrupy and thickened liquids are not). Generally, two tablespoons of thickener powder added to four ounces of liquid will produce a "honey" consistency. Using a measuring spoon and cup to thicken liquids will yield the most consistent results. Although any liquid can be thickened, some are more palatable when thickened (for example, orange juice) than others (like water). A speech therapist can provide specific instructions for how to adjust the amount of thickener needed for various liquids. Liquids thickened with cornstarch tend to continue to thicken further when left to stand—a factor that should be considered when planning a meal. Hot liquids tend to thicken faster than cold ones. Pre-thickened juices such as Resource are available commercially and are more convenient (though more expensive) than thickening liquids at home. These juices are generally supplied with a "nectar" consistency and must be further thickened for some individuals.

Some people find modified diets unappealing and so may not eat or drink sufficient amounts. Providing sufficient variety and ensuring that food is presented in an appealing fashion can go a long way toward improving the lives of people on severely restricted diets.

The social aspects of eating are very important. Many of our interactions, gatherings, and celebrations are focused around food and eating. Food shopping and preparation also have important social roles. Despite requiring a special diet, stroke survivors with dysphagia should be encouraged to participate in eating with family, and should sit at the same table as everyone else during holiday meals and other festive occasions.

Feeding Tubes

For many people with dysphagia, eating is not safe or is very limited initially. In these cases, alternative means of providing nutrition, fluids, and medications are needed. Intravenous fluids can provide a reliable and rapid way to restore fluids to someone who has become dehydrated or who can't take fluids safely by mouth. Standard intravenous fluids provide only minimal nutrition, however, and are not suitable for long-term nutritional support. In special circumstances, complete nutrition can be provided intravenously. This form of nutrition is known as total parenteral nutrition (or TPN). This method of providing nutrition carries a greater risk of complications than a feeding tube, and therefore is generally reserved for individuals who cannot eat and who have medical reasons preventing the use of a feeding tube. It is rarely appropriate for someone with post-stroke dysphagia.

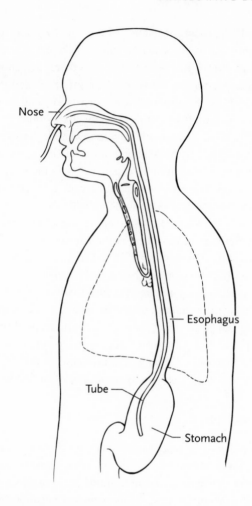

FIGURE 16.2   *Nasogastric tube.*
The nasogastric tube is inserted through the nose, down through the throat,
and into the stomach.

The most common initial method for feeding patients who are unable
to swallow safely is a nasogastric tube. The NG tube is placed through the
nose and passes through the back of the throat and down the esophagus
into the stomach (see Figure 16.2). These tubes have the advantage of being easily placed, and are an effective method to provide both food and

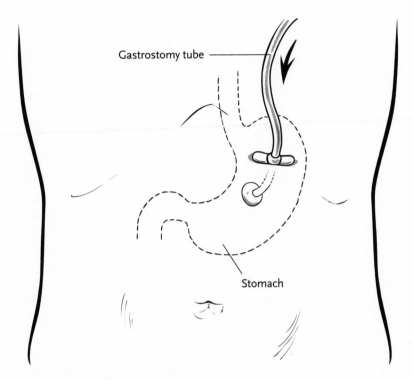

FIGURE 16.3   *Gastrostomy tube.*
One end of the gastrostomy tube is located in the stomach, and the other
end is outside the abdominal wall.

liquids. They do have a tendency to become dislodged, however, which
may lead to the need for frequent replacement. Because of their location,
they can be irritating, and some individuals have trouble tolerating them.
This is a particular problem for someone who is confused after a stroke.
For such an individual, a tube in the nose can be both irritating and easily removed, and thus he may pull out the tube repeatedly. This can lead
to the need to restrain the person's hands to prevent him from pulling
out the tube—certainly not an atmosphere very conducive to rehabilitation!

An alternative to an NG tube is a gastrostomy tube, sometimes termed
a G-tube or a PEG. These tubes are placed directly through the abdominal wall into the stomach (see Figure 16.3). Although placement of a G-

tube involves a minor surgical procedure, these tubes are often preferable to NG tubes for individuals with stroke who will require feeding
through a tube for an extended period. G-tubes are more comfortable for
the patient, since they do not go through the nose and are not located
near the face. They are also better secured than NG tubes and less likely
to become accidentally or intentionally dislodged.

Another, related type of tube is the jejunostomy tube, or J-tube. The jejunum is the first part of the small intestine, which begins shortly after
the stomach. Jejunostomy tubes can either be placed directly in the jejunum surgically or threaded through the stomach into the jejunum, in
which case they are known as GJ-tubes. Some physicians prefer J-tubes
to G-tubes, with the belief that they are less likely to cause reflux and possible pneumonia (see below). This issue remains undecided, and there is
not yet a consensus among physicians as to which type of tube is preferable. The disadvantages of a J-tube include a more difficult procedure for
placement, and the limited ability of the jejunum to accommodate large
amounts of tube feeding at once. Thus individuals with J-tubes may require continuous tube feeding, rather than several large tube feedings
during the course of a day.

Individuals receiving tube feedings can also aspirate those tube feedings as a result of vomiting or reflux. In reflux, the "valve" at the bottom
of the esophagus (known as the "lower esophageal sphincter") may not
function properly, allowing stomach contents to head back up toward the
mouth. When this happens, a person with dysphagia may not be able
to swallow this material properly and may aspirate it instead. Concern
about reflux is one of the reasons some physicians prefer jejunostomy
tubes to gastrostomy tubes, since the jejunostomy tube provides the
feeding further down the intestinal tract, beyond the stomach. This reduces the amount of material in the stomach and may prevent reflux
and possible aspiration. Whether this is an important enough difference
to justify placing J-tubes instead of G-tubes in all patients with stroke-
related dysphagia remains controversial. Family members can help prevent aspiration due to reflux by making certain that tube feedings are
provided when the stroke survivor is sitting or has the head of the bed elevated by at least thirty degrees. Once the patient is home, it may be necessary to obtain a hospital bed so that the head of the bed can be elevated.
Stroke survivors should not be put in a flat position or go to sleep imme-

diately after a tube feeding, but should instead maintain a sitting or partially upright position for at least one to two hours after feeding to reduce
the risk of reflux and aspiration.

Nutrition via a feeding tube is generally given with a standard nutritional liquid. Examples of such liquids include Ensure, Jevity, Ultracal,
and many others. These tube feedings are formulated to provide complete nutrition for extended periods. Some are palatable and come in different flavors; often these can also be used as oral nutritional supplements. Others are not intended for oral use and, though not dangerous,
are unlikely to be tasted more than once. There are special tube-feeding
formulations for individuals with diabetes (Glucerna), kidney disease
(Magnacal Renal), and pulmonary disease (Pulmocare), among others.
Some tube feedings contain dietary fiber to aid with normal digestive-
tract functioning and prevent constipation.

In the home setting, foods can also be liquified and put through a feeding tube. Although the person receiving the tube feeding can't taste the
food, she and her family may prefer a more "natural" diet. Care should be
taken that the foods are sufficiently liquified and sufficiently thinned
with water to flow easily through the tube. This type of feeding is not advisable through nasogastric tubes, since these can clog very easily.

Despite the fact that the commercially available feeding supplements
are liquid, they do not contain enough water for most people over the
course of a day. For this reason, extra water should be either mixed with
the tube feedings or given separately throughout the day. Typically, at
least a quart of extra water should be provided through the tube each day.
In hot weather, or if someone has a fever and has been sweating, extra
water should be given through the tube to prevent dehydration. Thirst
may not be a reliable indicator of insufficient fluid intake, particularly in
an elderly stroke survivor. One of the easiest ways for a family member to
determine if someone is receiving enough water through his tube is to
check urine production. If the person is only producing small amounts
of dark urine, he is not receiving enough water; if the urine is light-colored and of normal amount, then he is most likely receiving sufficient
water. Other clues to inadequate fluid intake are dry mouth and reduced
sweating.

Tube feedings are commonly given as a continuous infusion in the
hospital. In other words, a special pump is used to regulate the flow of

the tube feedings, so that a certain amount is given each hour. This technique is sometimes used at home, too, but it tends to be inconvenient owing to the need for the stroke survivor to be attached to a feeding pump. More commonly, the feedings will be changed to "bolus" feedings, in which the supplements are given several times a day in larger amounts—more akin to three or four meals a day. This is more convenient and also avoids the need for a special pump to regulate the speed of the feedings. If the feedings are given too quickly, they may cause stomach upset and even vomiting. If this happens, the tube feeds should be given more slowly to give the stomach time to adjust to the supplements.

Care of the G-tube "site" (where it enters through the skin) at home is primarily directed at keeping the area clean. Taking a cotton swab moistened with sterile saline and wiping away any accumulated mucous or crusted material daily is usually sufficient. If the amount of drainage seems excessive or if there is an increasing amount of redness around the site, consult a nurse or physician, since local infections can occasionally occur.

DURATION OF TUBE FEEDING

How long will a feeding tube be in place? Duration varies, depending on the severity of the swallowing problem. In most cases, swallowing improves substantially after stroke, and the feeding tube can be removed in a matter of weeks or months after its placement. In some strokes, however, more severe swallowing problems can occur, and a feeding tube may be required permanently. This is more common in older individuals, in individuals who have had more than one stroke, and in those with substantial cognitive limitations. Gastrostomy and jejunostomy tubes can be left in place indefinitely, whereas NG tubes tend to require periodic replacement. Removal of a nasogastric tube by a healthcare provider is very easy, as it simply slides out. G-tubes and J-tubes come in different varieties with different methods of removal. Most are removed by a physician at the bedside without any special procedure, however. If a feeding tube comes out unexpectedly, it should promptly be replaced by a medical professional. The "hole" for a gastrostomy or jejunostomy tube can close in a matter of hours, requiring a surgical procedure for replacement.

For the majority of people with feeding tubes who are transitioning from tube feeding to oral feeding, there is a period of overlap when they gradually increase their oral intake but still receive tube feeding. The decision of when to remove a tube depends on several factors. The primary factors determining this decision are the intake of adequate calories, protein, and fluids. Some individuals will be able to eat sufficient amounts of purees and thickened liquids to meet their caloric and other nutritional needs, but may have trouble drinking enough. In these situations, a feeding tube may be needed primarily for extra fluids.

When deciding whether or not to remove a feeding tube, it is important to consider the time and effort involved in eating. Some individuals are physically capable of eating enough to sustain themselves, but this process is so time-consuming and laborious that it takes up their entire day and is not pleasurable or practical. In these cases, it is reasonable for tube feeding and eating to continue in parallel as long as necessary or desired. Having a feeding tube does not preclude eating, and some people do best when maintaining a feeding tube to ensure adequate nutrition and fluid intake, while focusing on eating primarily for pleasure.

Ethical Dilemmas

Stuart is a sixty-two-year-old single Vietnam veteran who has been living alone for many years and runs his own car-repair business. He is hospitalized with a brainstem stroke resulting in severe dysphagia. He reluctantly accepts the placement of a gastrostomy tube early in his hospitalization but is becoming increasingly frustrated by his inability to resume eating. He informs his rehabilitation treatment team that he intends to stop his tube feeding and begin eating again, whether they feel that it is safe or not. Although his rehabilitation team accepts his right to make his own decisions, they are very concerned that he will develop pneumonia, and so they attempt to enlist the help of Stuart's niece, his only close family. His niece is distraught over the thought of her uncle's developing pneumonia and possibly even dying, and she spends several hours trying to understand his reasons for wanting to resume eating. What will happen if Stuart starts eating and aspirates? What should his niece do? What about the rehabilitation team—should they let him eat?

In the end, Stuart's niece works with the rehabilitation team to reach a compromise with Stuart—he will begin eating, even though this is contrary to medical advice, but he will eat only limited amounts and only with the assistance of a speech therapist. He will keep his G-tube for the time being, with an agreement that the team will reassess his progress in a few weeks. Stuart resumes eating gradually and develops an episode of pneumonia that is successfully treated with antibiotics. In spite of this problem, he continues to eat and eventually manages to have the G-tube removed, at which point he resumes a modified diet.

Stuart's case illustrates the need to consider each individual's personal perspective and preferences. While some people wish to minimize their medical risks and follow all the treatment recommendations of the rehabilitation team, others prefer to accept some risk consistent with their own values and priorities. It is important for family members to participate in this decision-making process, but to respect the wishes of the person who has to live with the impact of the choices he makes—the stroke survivor himself.

17

Pain and Muscle Spasms

Andrea is a thirty-five-year-old woman who has had a stroke related to systemic lupus erythematosus. As a result, she has severe weakness of her left side. Her left shoulder starts hurting about ten days after her stroke, and her physician notes that she has shoulder "subluxation." She is taught to support her shoulder using a lapboard and pillows in bed, and is given a sling by her physical therapist to use during walking. Despite this treatment, her shoulder pain persists and is interfering with her rehabilitation. She undergoes a shoulder injection with methylprednisolone (Depo-medrol), which results in gradual improvement of her symptoms. Although her subluxation persists, her pain does not recur. Why did she develop a painful shoulder? Could this have been prevented?

Pain after Stroke

Pain is a relatively uncommon complication of stroke, but it can be severe when it does occur. Pain after a stroke falls into two broad categories—central pain syndromes, in which the injury to the brain causes the perception of pain in the body; and peripheral pain, in which the pain is caused by a stimulus in the body that indirectly results from the stroke. An example of the latter is shoulder pain after stroke.

Central Pain

Central pain can occur after a stroke affecting the thalamus, a central relay station in the brain that helps transmit sensation from the body to the brain. The most severe thalamic pain syndromes are usually associated with severe loss of normal sensation (see Chapter 12). Some have suggested that thalamic pain syndromes occur because the brain is unable to receive normal sensation from the affected side of the body and so "substitutes" abnormal (pain) sensations on its own to "fill in the gap." Central pain varies in quality but is most commonly described as burning. Central pain syndromes can also develop after strokes in other parts of the brain, but they are less common and less well characterized than thalamic pain syndromes.

Treatment for central pain syndromes involves a variety of medications, though it is often hard to predict which medication will be most effective for a given person. Anticonvulsant (antiseizure) medications have been among the most effective treatments, with Neurontin (gabapentin) a common first choice, followed by Tegretol (carbamezapine), Dilantin (phenytoin), and others. Tricyclic antidepressant medications such as Elavil (amitryptiline), Norpramin (desipramine), and others are also useful for some individuals with central pain after stroke. Conventional pain medications such as Tylenol (acetaminophen), Motrin (ibuprofen), and Oxycontin (oxycodone) are generally not as helpful in this condition, though some people do experience relief with them.

Peripheral Pain

The most common pain problems after a stroke do not directly result from the damage to the brain, but rather are related to problems in the arms or legs that occur because of weakness or abnormal muscle tone.

SHOULDER PAIN

Among the most common of these problems is pain in the weak shoulder. Shoulder pain after stroke is most often seen when shoulder "subluxation" occurs. In shoulder subluxation, the weakened shoulder muscles are unable to hold the shoulder joint in its usual position. Normally, the shoulder joint relies on its muscles to keep it in the correct position. With these muscles unable to perform their usual job owing to weakness from a stroke, the upper arm bone, known as the humerus, tends to hang down. This causes a gap between the bones in the shoulder. The gap can be seen and felt, allowing physicians and therapists to identify the presence of a shoulder subluxation. Although it is not entirely clear how shoulder subluxation causes shoulder pain, it appears that the tendons, ligaments, muscles, and joint capsule are all stretched by the subluxation, resulting in pain. The basic treatment for this problem is to support the shoulder so that it can be maintained in its normal position. This involves using pillows while in bed, a cushioned tray when seated in a wheelchair, and a sling while walking. Fortunately, most people gradually accommodate to the subluxation and their pain resolves. They can usually eliminate the use of arm supports and slings over time. Some people with subluxation never experience pain. Others may have little detectable subluxation but will nonetheless experience shoulder pain. In a few cases, the shoulder subluxation triggers inflammation of the rotator cuff muscles and tendons, leading to persistent pain that is not resolved with the use of arm supports. In these cases, an injection of a cortisone-like medication (such as the corticosteroid Depo-Medrol) into the shoulder region may be helpful.

WRIST AND HAND PAIN

Another common area for pain after stroke is the hand and wrist. As with shoulder pain, pain in these areas seems to be related to positioning difficulties that develop as a result of muscle weakness. Abnormal muscle tone, as discussed below, can contribute to abnormal positioning at these joints. As with shoulder pain, these problems are best treated by improving positioning of the involved area(s). Wrist or combined wrist-hand splints are commonly employed as a means of improving positioning of the wrist and fingers. These splints are typically worn either during the day or at night, though usually not twenty-four hours per day. A wrist-hand splint worn primarily for positioning will often be used at night, to allow maximum movement during the day. A wrist splint that is used to stabilize the wrist for functional tasks is commonly worn during the day.

COMPLEX REGIONAL PAIN SYNDROME
(REFLEX SYMPATHETIC DYSTROPHY)

Occasionally, some individuals will develop persistent severe shoulder and wrist-hand pain that does not appear to be due to local factors alone (such as subluxation), and is not believed to be due to a central pain syndrome resulting directly from the stroke. This condition, complex regional pain syndrome (CRPS), is also known as reflex sympathetic dystrophy (RSD), or shoulder-hand syndrome. The causes of this syndrome are still hotly debated, though its frequency after stroke appears to be relatively low with appropriate rehabilitation. An important aspect of this syndrome is the development of hypersensitivity of the affected areas. Stroke survivors with CRPS sometimes describe even light touch of the affected area as painful. This hypersensitivity leads the affected person to avoid any touch or movement of the arm. Unfortunately, this natural protective response may actually worsen the problem of hypersensitivity.

Prevention is the key to this syndrome, and it consists of a regular program of stretching the arm and using it for exercises as much as possible. The more the arm is massaged and manipulated, the less likely it is to develop RSD. When symptoms suggestive of RSD develop, the best treatment is to increase the use of massage and range-of-motion exercises. This desensitization therapy prevents the worsening of the hypersensitivity, helps to reverse it, and is the cornerstone of treatment. Medications are sometimes used as well, and include the same medications discussed above for central pain syndromes. In severe or persistent cases, evaluation by a pain specialist is recommended, and treatment may include specialized injections.

CARPAL TUNNEL SYNDROME

Stroke survivors sometimes develop tingling pain and loss of feeling in the "good" hand as a result of carpal tunnel syndrome. This condition is particularly common in individuals who rely on a cane to help them walk. The pain and numbness are caused by damage to one of the major nerves in the wrist (the median nerve) as a result of putting extra pressure on the hand and wrist. Treatments include changing the type of cane or handgrip, using wrist splints, and/or receiving injections to relieve inflammation. In severe or persistent cases, surgery of the wrist can provide more room for the nerve, alleviate pain, and prevent further damage to the nerve.

KNEE PAIN

Knee pain can occur in the weak leg after stroke owing to changes in the normal walking pattern. An altered gait can cause the knee to "snap back" (also known as knee hyperextension), resulting in pain and swelling. Failure to correct this abnormal motion can lead to permanent damage and premature arthritis of the knee joint. An ankle or knee brace and appropriate orthopedic shoes are the treatment of choice to protect the knee from this mechanical stress.

HEADACHE

Headache can occur at the time of a stroke, though it is usually absent or mild in ischemic stroke. Headache is quite common in cerebral hemorrhages, however, and may be quite severe in some cases. Typically, headache resulting from a stroke gradually resolves over time. Analgesics such as Tylenol and Percocet are the usual first-line treatments. Persistent headache after stroke is unusual and should be evaluated by a physician.

HIP OR BACK PAIN

Hip and back pain are not very common early on after a stroke but can develop over time as a late side effect. This type of pain is usually due to altered walking patterns that put new stresses on the hips and back and can cause muscular or arthritic pain. A careful reevaluation of a person's gait by a rehabilitation professional experienced in stroke care (physiatrist or physical therapist) may be helpful in developing a treatment plan.

Spasticity

Pamela had a stroke six months ago, with severe weakness of her right arm. Initially her arm was very limp and tended to hang down and flop about. Unfortunately, though Pamela's leg strength and walking have improved substantially, her arm remains severely affected by the stroke, with minimal movement. She has noticed that over the past few months her arm has become more and more bent at the elbow, and her hand has gradually become clenched into a fist. She notes some redness in her hand from the pressure of her fingernails on her palm, and she is concerned that she will have difficulty getting a blouse on if her arm becomes more bent and difficult to straighten. Her physician and occupational therapist have advised her to wear a nighttime splint to hold her wrist and fingers in proper position, as well as to perform daily stretching exercises. Pamela follows these instructions and finds that though the tightness persists, it doesn't get any worse and is controlled with the splint and stretching exercises. What causes this muscle stiffness? Can it be prevented? What treatments are available?

Weakness is one of the hallmark features of stroke, but paradoxically, stroke can also lead to increased muscle tone and stiffness. This increase in muscle tone is known as "spasticity." Spasticity after a stroke is usually manifested as muscle tightness or stiffness, but it can also result in uncontrolled muscle spasms. Rhythmic ankle spasms, known as "clonus," are quite common after stroke. Although spasticity can affect any muscle or group of muscles, it tends to be particularly problematic in a few areas, such as the elbow, wrist, fingers, and ankle. Since this increase in muscle tone is not under a person's conscious control, it can, in some cases, interfere with comfort or function.

Pamela's experience is fairly typical. While there are exceptions, spasticity generally occurs in a stroke survivor with severe weakness and little control over a weak arm or leg. It usually develops gradually over a period of weeks to months, though occasionally it will be present almost immediately after a stroke. In many cases it seems that the earlier spasticity develops, the more severe it will become. Still, in most cases, no treatment beyond proper positioning (for example, with a splint) and stretching is required. Some of my patients have managed to control even severe spasticity for many years with careful attention to regular stretching and positioning.

It is very important to recognize that spasticity is not necessarily a bad thing, and it usually does not require medical treatment. Moreover, it often helps substitute for the function of weak muscles after stroke, and can actually help people function better. The most common example of this is spasticity affecting the leg after stroke. In most cases, spasticity at the hip and knee joints tends to keep the leg straight and stiffened. This stiffness can allow someone without much muscle control in the leg to bear weight on the leg, and walk, even without exercising muscle control. Treatment that takes away this muscle spasticity may actually interfere with a person's ability to walk and so should not be undertaken.

It is also important to recognize that spasticity does not usually "mask" underlying muscle control. Some stroke survivors (and some physicians too) may be under the impression that a person's arm (or other limb) would "work better" if the spasticity were reduced. Although spasticity can be the limiting factor in the use of a limb after stroke, this is rarely the case. Usually the limiting factor is the loss of muscle control, and the spasticity is not truly responsible for the functional limitations. Overall, one should approach treatment for spasticity thoughtfully. Only a minority of individuals with spasticity after stroke actually require treatment. For the rest, stretching and the use of appropriate splints are generally sufficient and most appropriate.

Spasticity Treatments

In some cases, spasticity proceeds to the point where more intensive treatment is needed. This situation usually arises when the spasticity is causing pain or substantial difficulty with positioning. When further treatment is needed, there are several options. One option is oral medications, several of which are available to treat spasticity. Each of these medications has its advantages and disadvantages, and trial and error is often necessary to select the best medication for a given person. Baclofen (Lioresal) is usually my first choice for an oral medication when treating spasticity after stroke. Tizanidine (Zanaflex) is a newer medication with similar overall benefits to baclofen but better results in some people. Valium (diazepam) and related medications such as Klonopin (clonazepam) are alternative choices, with effects similar to, though perhaps a little less effective than, baclofen. All these oral medications suffer from certain limitations: all are sedating and may worsen any cognitive problems or fatigue that a person is experiencing after stroke. These side effects often limit the dose that a person can tolerate, and this dose may not be sufficient to control the spasticity. Nor are oral medications for spasticity capable of specifically targeting the muscles that are causing the symptoms—in fact, they affect all the muscles of the body equally. Dantrolene (Dantrium) is another oral medication used for spasticity after stroke, and though generally considered less sedating than the other medications mentioned above, also affects all muscles equally. Moreover, dantrolene and tizanidine (and to a lesser extent, baclofen) can all cause liver abnormalities in a small number of people, and monitoring of blood tests is recommended.

Botox: From Food Poisoning to Wrinkle Reduction

Botulinum toxin is an interesting substance and a surprising treatment in some ways. It is made by a bacteria, *clostridium botulinum,* and is the toxin that causes botulism (a severe form of food poisoning) in cases of improperly canned mushrooms and other foods. In food-related poisoning, a large dose is absorbed by the body, causing weakness of all muscles, with paralysis and inability to breath. When purified and injected in small doses into a muscle, however, the toxin causes only local weakness and is a well-tolerated and safe medicine. In another interesting "wrinkle," botulinum toxin type A (Botox) is now increasingly used to treat facial wrinkles. Here too, it works by weakening selected muscles and preventing them from crinkling the forehead, causing "crows' feet" and other age-related imperfections.

Another treatment approach for spasticity is the use of local injections. These include botulinum toxin, phenol, and alcohol. Injection of the nerve(s) or muscle(s) most affected by spasticity allows reduction of spasticity where it is causing the most symptoms, while avoiding the side effects of sedation or generalized weakness seen with oral medications. As a result, injections are often used as an initial treatment for spasticity after stroke, even before oral medications. This is particularly appropriate if the spasticity is localized to a small number of muscles.

Botulinum toxin is available in the United States in two distinct varieties: botulinum toxin type A, known as Botox, and botulinum toxin type B, known as Myobloc. While Botox has been more extensively studied for the treatment of spasticity after stroke, both medications appear to be effective for this problem. Botulinum toxin prevents the nerve impulses from reaching the muscle and is given as one or several injections directly into the muscle. Botulinum toxin is quite safe when administered in appropriate amounts and generally works well. The two major drawbacks to its use are that it is quite expensive (medication costs alone for an injection for spasticity may be more than $1,200) and the effects typically last for only three months. Since spasticity after stroke can be a lifelong problem, treatment with botulinum toxin may become an expensive and time-consuming process. Its benefits include safety, complete reversibility after three months, and ease of injection.

Another option for treatment of spasticity is the injection of phenol. Phenol works by destroying some of the nerve fibers to the muscle. It is a somewhat caustic substance and can cause swelling and/or pain when injected. There are several methods of injection. The safest method involves targeting the smaller branches of the nerves that connect to the muscle. This technique, known as a "motor point block," is generally well tolerated but more painful than botulinum toxin injection, which is nearly painless. In a small number of cases phenol can cause a persistent unpleasant burning sensation known as a dysesthesia. Rarely, long-term pain can occur as a complication of phenol injection, though this is seldom seen when the injection is administered by an experienced physician using the appropriate technique. (Note that the risks of phenol injection are greater when larger nerves are injected instead of the smaller nerves in a motor point block.) Phenol differs from botulinim toxin in several important ways: Unlike botulinum toxin, phenol is inexpensive. It is also longer lasting, with the effects typically being felt for about six months. Also, unlike botulinum toxin, the effects of phenol injection are cumulative if repeated, and one or two injections are usually sufficient for prolonged benefits. Phenol administration requires a physician trained and experienced in its use, and may not be available in some areas. Botulinum toxin is less technically demanding to inject and is more broadly available. Concentrated alcohol may also be injected in a manner similar to phenol, though it may cause more pain when injected and is less widely used in the United States.

In severe cases of widespread spasticity, another treatment has been found effective, though it is more invasive. This treatment is called "intrathecal baclofen" and involves the placement of a self-contained pump under the skin to provide a constant dose of baclofen. The hockey-puck-sized pump is connected to a catheter (tube) that goes under the skin and delivers the baclofen to the fluid around the spinal cord. This treatment delivers a small amount of baclofen right to where it has its beneficial effects, specifically, the spinal cord. Because this treatment delivers the medication precisely where it is needed, it allows someone to receive a large benefit from a small amount of medication, and avoids the side effects of fatigue or cognitive dysfunction commonly seen with oral baclofen. The effects of intrathecal baclofen are most dramatic in the legs and intermediate in the arms. There is usually little or no effect on any spasticity impacting the head or neck.

Intrathecal baclofen has been used with considerable success in other disorders complicated by spasticity, such as spinal cord injury and multiple sclerosis. Its use for stroke has been more limited. Very few cases of spasticity after stroke are severe enough to justify this type of treatment, and most cases are responsive to less invasive treatments. Risks of this treatment include infections of the device, mechanical pump failures, dislodged or blocked catheters, and over- or under-dosage owing to programming errors. The pumps need to be refilled in a brief office procedure every one to three months. The pumps themselves require replacement when the battery runs down, after approximately seven years. Intrathecal baclofen treatment is quite expensive but is generally covered by insurance companies when medically indicated.

18

Equipment and Home Environment

Michelle's family is preparing for her return home after a stroke at age sixty-nine. Although Michelle has made good progress in her rehabilitation, she still requires the use of a wheelchair much of the time and needs help getting in and out of the bathroom. Michelle's daughter will be staying in her mother's apartment with her initially, until Michelle is able to manage independently. Her daughter wants to make certain she has the appropriate equipment available for Michelle at home, but she is also concerned that the apartment they will be sharing is small and already a bit cluttered. How can her daughter make certain that the apartment is appropriately set up for Michelle, and that the right equipment has been obtained?

Making a home environment safe and accessible plays an important role in the stroke survivor's successful reintegration into the community. Often, as in Michelle's case, the physical constraints of a particular home can limit the success of this effort. For example, a third-floor walk-up apartment will never be optimally accessible for a stroke survivor who requires a wheelchair. Personal preference plays a substantial role in home arrangements as well, including the selection of equipment. Some stroke survivors may prefer not to use equipment to assist in a task if they can still manage the task without it, even if the equipment would reduce the time and effort required. Physical and occupational therapists, often in conjunction with a physician specializing in physical medicine and rehabilitation, can provide guidance for families considering home modifications or obtaining equipment for a stroke survivor.

Creating a Safe Home Environment

Creating a safe environment at home depends on the specific issues facing a stroke survivor. If a stroke survivor has poor judgment owing to cognitive effects of the stroke but is physically mobile, the key issues may be preventing access to dangerous areas or activities. Keeping the car keys in a secure location, preventing access to the stove, or securing a basement workshop area may be necessary in some cases. A careful discussion with the rehabilitation team before return home can usually identify potential risks to the cognitively impaired stroke survivor in the home environment.

Establishing a home environment that is safe for a stroke survivor who requires a wheelchair or uses a cane to walk is a very common scenario. Carpeting often makes the use of wheeled devices, such as wheelchairs and walkers, very difficult, and it may need to be removed. Generally, thick carpeting presents a greater challenge than thin carpeting. Area or throw rugs present a hazard for almost anyone with mobility problems after stroke, since the edges can trip someone who has difficulty walking and make wheelchair use difficult.

Other hazards to walking or wheelchair use in the home include long electrical cords or extension cords. A foot, wheelchair, cane, or walker can catch on the cord, causing a fall. These cords should be kept out of areas where walking occurs. In general, a cluttered environment is more difficult for a stroke survivor to negotiate than an open area. Coffee tables, free-standing lamps, excessively cluttered furniture, and any other obstacles to easy movement in a straight line can make mobility difficult for a stroke survivor and increase the risk of falls.

Many homes have raised thresholds between rooms that can trip someone who has trouble walking or make wheelchair movement more difficult. In some cases, removal of these raised thresholds may be feasible and worth considering to enhance safety.

Narrow doorways can present an important obstacle to wheelchair users, and one that may influence the choice of wheelchair. A standard wheelchair requires a doorway that is at least thirty-two inches wide. Older homes may have narrower doorways, and a standard wheelchair may not fit through them. Narrower wheelchairs are available, though many stroke survivors cannot comfortably fit in them. Doorways should be measured before ordering a wheelchair to avoid any unpleasant surprises when using the wheelchair in the home.

Bedrooms

The height and type of bed can affect a stroke survivor's mobility and independence at home. Some beds are higher or lower than standard height and can be difficult to get in and out of. Measuring the height of the bed and sharing this information with the rehabilitation team can ensure that the stroke survivor has appropriate training getting in and out of bed before returning home. Some beds are less firm than others and may interfere with mobility. Waterbeds in particular may be especially challenging for a mobility-impaired stroke survivor. Generally, firmer beds create a more stable surface and make movement in and out of the bed easier.

A few stroke survivors benefit from the use of a hospital bed. These are generally individuals with severely limited mobility who may require the head of the bed to be elevated for tube feedings or other medical needs. Hospital beds are large and may be difficult to fit into a small room. Insurance frequently covers hospital bed rentals when appropriate documentation of medical need is provided by the physician.

Some stroke survivors can manage fairly well in a regular bed but have trouble rolling or turning in bed as a result of weakness. A bed rail can be attached to the bed to assist the person when rolling or moving about the bed. This device is inexpensive and easily attaches to most beds.

In cases of severe mobility limitations the caregiver may not be able to help the stroke survivor get out of bed and into a wheelchair. Sometimes a simple device known as a sliding board can provide a smooth surface allowing a person literally to slide from the bed into the wheelchair or the reverse. Although this device usually still requires the assistance of a caregiver, it reduces the physical demands on the caregiver considerably.

In cases where a sliding board is not feasible or insufficient, a device known as a "Hoyer lift" can be used ("Hoyer" is a brand name; several other manufacturers sell similar devices). These lifts have a fabric harness that is placed underneath the stroke survivor while he is in the bed and then attached to a sturdy metal hoist. These lifts come in both manual versions, in which an arm crank is used to lift the person into the air, and electric versions when the arm crank is not feasible. Once the person has been lifted into the air with the Hoyer lift, he can be swung over the wheelchair and then lowered into the chair. The fabric harness stays underneath the person while he is in the wheelchair, and the process is reversed when he returns to bed. Hoyer lifts require a relatively large room and may not fit in some bedrooms. A device similar to a Hoyer lift (Guldmann lift—see Appendix p. 245 under "Guldmann, Inc.") can be permanently installed on the ceiling of the room. Although this option is more expensive and less portable than a traditional Hoyer lift, it can be more convenient and requires less space.

Bathrooms

Bathrooms are one of the most challenging rooms in the home for many stroke survivors to negotiate. They are usually small, crowded spaces, and often have wet, slippery, and hard surfaces. A variety of equipment and modifications exist to make a bathroom easier for a stroke survivor to access and utilize safely.

Grab bars are metal or plastic bars attached to the walls of the bathroom in strategic locations to help a stroke survivor get on and off the toilet, as well as manage in the shower more safely. These bars should be professionally installed to ensure that they are adequately anchored to the wall.

Tub benches and shower chairs allow a person to shower while seated in order to avoid falls. Tub benches are used when a bathroom has a showerhead located above a bathtub, whereas a shower chair is used for a stall shower. These devices come in a variety of sizes and variations—an occupational therapist can assist in choosing the most appropriate one.

After a stroke some people have difficulty rising from a standard-height toilet owing to weakness or arthritis. A raised toilet seat allows a person easier access on and off the toilet. Some raised toilet seats come with built-in grab bars that may provide further assistance if needed.

Leaning over to wash feet or other difficult-to-reach areas can be hazardous for a person with impaired balance after a stroke. Long-handled shower sponges are an inexpensive device that can help a person bathe more independently.

In some cases, a bathroom cannot be made safe and accessible for a stroke survivor, or is on the wrong floor in the house for someone who cannot negotiate stairs. A bedside commode is the answer for some people and can allow them to retain as much independence as possible. Commodes come in a variety of shapes and sizes, including extra-wide for larger individuals, with padded seats, and with drop-arms to allow easier transfers on and off the commode.

Stairs

Stairs are a major barrier for many stroke survivors. Installation of handrails on both sides of a staircase can help make stairs more accessible. For outdoor stairs, a ramp may be a suitable alternative. Ramps can be permanent or temporary and movable—the latter may be appropriate for an infrequently used set of stairs or where a permanent ramp is not feasible. Ramps that are too steep may be difficult to negotiate and even dangerous. Permanent ramps should be installed by someone knowledgeable to ensure an appropriate incline and suitable nonslip surface.

Creative approaches are sometimes needed for stroke survivors to manage stairs safely. These can include descending backward or sitting down and "bumping" down on the buttocks. A physical therapist can provide training in managing stairs and can help devise solutions for specific situations.

In some cases, a motorized stair lift may be the best option. These systems require professional installation and are expensive, but they can provide a higher level of independence for a stroke survivor. It is important for family members to realize that these lifts are not appropriate for every stroke survivor who cannot manage the stairs. In particular, the stroke survivor using the lift must have sufficient balance and trunk control to stay safely seated while ascending or descending on the lift. Otherwise he may fall and sustain injury.

Kitchen and Dining Area

The kitchen and dining area commonly serve as the social hub of a home and are where a large percentage of waking hours are spent. Food preparation is a task that often has important personal meaning beyond merely putting food on the table. For many people, preparing meals helps define their role in the family. The ability to participate in food preparation and dining with other family members is an important goal for many stroke survivors.

In order to ensure safe food preparation, family members need to consider the presence of any cognitive limitations. Memory or attention deficits can lead to burns, kitchen fires, or worse. Occupational therapists commonly evaluate kitchen safety as part of their overall home-safety assessment, and they can provide guidance regarding a stroke survivor's safety in the kitchen. If in doubt, family members should provide adequate supervision until convinced that a stroke survivor can manage safely on his own.

Physical limitations in the kitchen can affect a variety of activities. Difficulty standing for prolonged periods can impair a person's ability to cook, so some stroke survivors may need to work from a wheelchair or kitchen chair to prevent fatigue. Carrying utensils and ingredients within the kitchen can be a challenge for someone with weakness on one side who requires a cane or walker. Special baskets are available that attach to these devices to help carry items safely while using a walking aid.

A variety of clever and inexpensive assistive devices are available to help the stroke survivor with food preparation. An occupational therapist can help identify appropriate devices and provide instruction in their use. Cutting boards with "spikes" to hold the food in place while it's being cut, weighted bowels and other implements that do not move while their contents are being mixed, and many other devices are available to help with one-handed food preparation. These devices can be ordered from catalogues and web sites (see Appendix for specifics).

Similarly, a variety of devices can assist with one-handed eating or with weakness or reduced coordination. Plates with a raised edge on one side to help "push" food onto a fork, weighted cups that resist tipping over, rocker knives for one-handed use, and other devices are widely available (see Figure 18.1).

Some stroke survivors have difficulty rising from couches or other low surfaces. Avoiding low, cushiony surfaces such as couches or lounge chairs and using firmer chairs with high seats are often sufficient to address this problem. A cushion can be added to a firm seat surface to raise the seat height somewhat. Devices are available to help people with im-

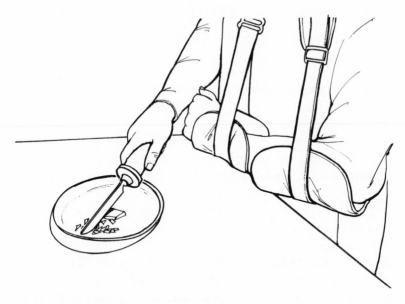

FIGURE 18.1 *Adapted plate and rocker knife.*
An adapted plate with a raised edge on one side allows food to be pushed
onto a fork or spoon; a rocker knife allows for one-handed cutting.

paired mobility rise from a chair, but they are only occasionally needed
by stroke survivors.

Car

Although we don't generally think of the car as part of the home, in many
ways it serves as a sort of mobile room for many people. Helping the
stroke survivor get in and out of a car is an important task for family
members to practice with the rehabilitation team before the return home
from the hospital. Most standard wheelchairs are foldable and easily
placed in the car by a caregiver. For wheelchair users traveling alone by
car, or users of nonfolding or power wheelchairs, transportation of the
wheelchair can present a challenge. Special lift devices are available to
help transport of these wheelchairs into a car.

Mobility Aids and Other Equipment

Wheelchairs

Many stroke survivors require the use of a wheelchair—some for only a short time, others for the indefinite future. Wheelchairs come in a dizzying array of varieties, and wheelchair vendors vary in their expertise in providing the best choice. Purchasing the wrong wheelchair can be an expensive and frustrating mistake, so obtaining expert guidance from a physical therapist, physiatrist, or other rehabilitation provider with experience in this area is well worth the effort.

Manual wheelchairs are the most commonly used type, and are relatively simple and portable. A standard manual wheelchair rental may be all that a stroke survivor needs, particularly if he is only using the wheelchair outside of the home for extended travel or visits to the mall. Lightweight wheelchairs are similar in structure and function to standard wheelchairs but are lighter in weight. For someone who will be propelling her own wheelchair for extended periods, a lightweight wheelchair is generally a good idea.

"Hemi" chairs are wheelchairs in which the seating platform is closer to the ground than usual. This allows someone to use his intact leg to help propel and steer the wheelchair, rather than using only his intact arm. These chairs are generally preferable to one-arm drive wheelchairs, which are sometimes used as an alternative. One-arm drive wheelchairs have two rims on the intact side, one of which is attached through the axle to the wheel on the opposite side of the wheelchair. By alternating use of the rims, the wheelchair occupant can control both wheels. In practice, most people find a hemi chair or a power wheelchair a better option, though some do find one-arm drive chairs useful.

Reclining wheelchairs have a back support that can be adjusted to tilt backward to varying angles. These chairs are useful for individuals with reduced trunk control, who may otherwise slump forward in the wheelchair. In more severe cases of reduced trunk control, a wheelchair in which the entire seating surface can rotate backward may be useful (for example, a "Tilt in Space" wheelchair). These wheelchairs are larger, heavier, and more expensive than standard wheelchairs but provide excellent support in these cases. Side supports can also be added to these wheelchairs for people who tend to slump to one side or the other.

People who cannot propel a manual chair sufficiently, or who need a wheelchair and are highly active, sometimes find a manual chair too fatiguing or too slow. For these stroke survivors, a power wheelchair (sometimes called an electric wheelchair) may provide a solution. Because of the size and power of these devices, users must be able to control them safely to avoid injury to themselves or others around them. People with cognitive, attentional, or perceptual problems may not be able to use these chairs safely. Power chairs are expensive, heavy, large, difficult to transport, need to be recharged regularly, and can break down. For these reasons, a manual chair is always needed as a backup. Family members contemplating obtaining a power wheelchair for their family member should consider how they will transport the wheelchair in and out of the home and in the car. Expert advice is particularly important when choosing a power wheelchair.

Scooters are a popular device often used as an alternative to a power wheelchair. Electric scooters are often less expensive, and may be perceived as less socially stigmatizing, than a power wheelchair. Scooters are generally three-wheeled and less mechanically stable than four-wheeled power wheelchairs. Scooters provide less trunk support than power wheelchairs, are less easily customized, and are thus not suitable as an alternative for many stroke survivors. For the partially ambulatory stroke survivor, however, a scooter may be a good choice.

A new type of power-assisted manual wheelchair, the iGLIDE, may be appropriate for selected individuals after stroke. This wheelchair can be used as a conventional manual wheelchair but also has a power-assisted mode that gives the user help propelling the wheelchair on difficult terrain (for example, grass or carpeting), uphill, or when fatigued. This type of wheelchair is designed for individuals who are able to use both arms to propel a wheelchair, and is thus suitable for only a selected group of stroke survivors.

Wheelchairs can be customized with a variety of additions to improve comfort and safety. Wheelchair cushions can protect against excessive pressure on the buttocks and can prevent sores from developing. For wheelchair users who spend extended periods in the chair, a padded solid seat bottom and/or seat back can provide greater support and comfort than a fabric sling design. For individuals who have difficulty reaching the brake levers, brake handle extenders make this task easier from an upright position. Seatbelts are often useful to protect against sliding out of the wheelchair. Lap trays can offer a convenient surface for eating or other activities in the wheelchair, and can provide support for a weak arm with shoulder subluxation. An arm board can provide similar support for a weak arm, without adding the bulk or restriction of a full lap tray.

RENT OR PURCHASE?

The decision to rent versus purchase a wheelchair depends on several factors. The first is the duration of the anticipated use. Is the wheelchair only going to be used for a transition period while walking continues to improve? If so, a wheelchair rental usually makes the most sense. For long-term use, a purchase may be more appropriate. Many wheelchairs can be obtained on a rent-purchase system, whereby the user owns the wheelchair after renting for a certain period of time. For specialized or customized wheelchairs, purchase may be the only option, as these chairs may not be available for rent.

Canes and Walkers

Many stroke survivors rely on canes or other ambulatory aids to help them walk safely. Canes come in several varieties, though they most commonly have one or four prongs on the bottom to help provide support (see Figure 18.2). Single-prong canes with expanded bases are also available and serve a similar purpose to multipronged canes. Generally, the wider the base of the cane, the more support it provides. Often, a person will progress from a wide-based four-pronged ("quad") cane to a small-based quad cane, and finally to a single cane.

Walkers are sometimes appropriate for stroke survivors, but many individuals cannot use them owing to weakness in one hand or arm that prevents them from gripping the walker sufficiently. Walkers may come with or without wheels—the former are easier to push forward but do not provide as much stability as the latter. Some walker-like de-

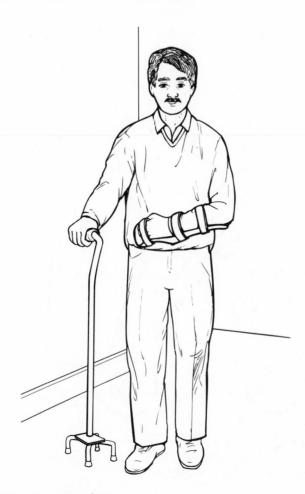

FIGURE 18.2   *Four-pronged cane.*
A four-pronged cane is a useful walking aid for stroke survivors with
weakness.

vices have four wheels and use handbrakes (similar to bicycle brakes).
These devices, known as "rollators," provide limited stability (see Figure 18.3).

Canes with broader sculpted handles may be easier for some individuals to grasp effectively. For people residing in colder climates, small "ice

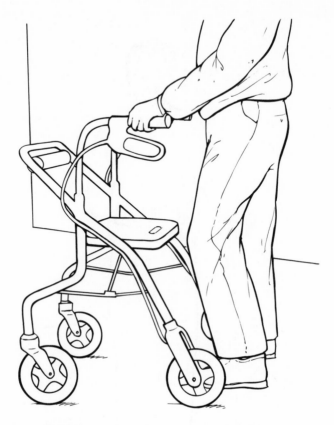

FIGURE 18.3   *Rollator.*
This rolling walker with handbrakes is suitable for individuals with good use
of both hands and a mild loss of balance.

grippers" can be attached to the bottom of the cane to provide extra trac-
tion in icy conditions.

Braces

Braces are frequently needed to help with walking after stroke. Most individuals needing a brace after a stroke will receive one that comes up to
the upper calf, known as an ankle-foot orthosis or AFO (see Figure 18.4).
AFOs are usually made of plastic and may be prefabricated, off-the-shelf
devices, or created from a custom mold of the leg. They come in varying

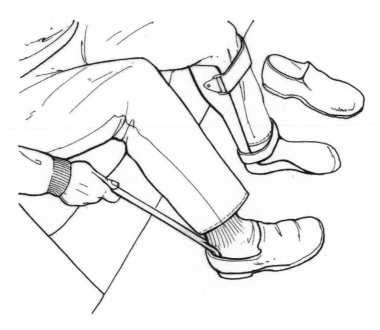

FIGURE 18.4 *Ankle foot orthosis (AFO) and dressing stick.*
An ankle foot orthosis (left foot) helps stroke survivors with ankle weakness
to walk. The multipurpose dressing stick, used here as a long-handled shoe
horn, helps with a variety of dressing tasks.

degrees of stiffness, depending on the degree of weakness and the presence or absence of abnormally increased muscle tone in the leg. AFOs
are generally worn over a cotton sock and fit inside the shoe. They are
usually worn inside of slacks, though they may be worn over tightly
fitting leggings or tights. Braces serve several purposes, including lifting
up the toes to prevent dragging, preventing twisting inward of the ankle,
and stabilizing the knee somewhat. AFOs with ankle hinges are useful
for selected individuals, though they tend to be a bit bulkier and less du-
rable than AFOs fabricated as a single piece.

Some individuals require metal braces instead of plastic, usually because of fluctuating ankle swelling, skin problems, or obesity. These
metal braces are riveted to special orthopedic shoes rather than inserted
into the shoe as an AFO. Occasionally, more substantial braces that
go above the knee are required; these are known as knee-ankle-foot

orthoses, or KAFOs. These braces are usually reserved for stroke survivors with severe knee-control problems.

Although most braces are fabricated from polypropylene (a translucent plastic) or metal, some newer braces are made from high-tech materials such as carbon fiber or Kevlar. All lower-extremity braces should be fitted by a qualified orthotist as prescribed by a knowledgeable physician.

Shoulder Supports

Stroke survivors with severe shoulder weakness and subluxation are often fitted with slings to support the arm and prevent or alleviate shoulder pain (see Figure 18.1). Slings are generally made from fabric and can be simple or elaborate. Simple, less restrictive slings are usually preferable to elaborate ones and are easier to put on and take off. Stroke survivors using slings should be certain to keep the affected arm flexible by removing the sling periodically each day and performing stretching exercises on the arm and hand. The shoulder pain resulting from subluxation tends to improve over time, and in many cases sling use can eventually be discontinued in consultation with the physician or therapist.

Splints

Splints are similar to braces; they are essentially devices to hold the affected limb in the desired position. Splints are commonly used for the wrist and hand to prevent the hand from losing range of motion and curling up into a fist. Wrist-hand splints are generally used either during the nighttime hours or during the daytime; the rest of the time the hand remains open. Removing the splint provides an opportunity to exercise and stretch the muscles and joints of the wrist and hand, as well as to give the skin a chance to air out. I generally advise nighttime splint use when possible, to encourage whatever functional use is possible during the daytime. Most splints are plastic and may be off-the-shelf or custom fabricated by an occupational therapist (see Figure 18.5). Sometimes fabric splints (with metal supports inside) are used to stabilize only the wrist, and leave the hand free for the stroke survivor to use functionally.

For people with increased muscle tone in the ankle, a nighttime ankle splint may be needed. These devices are usually prefabricated and serve to maintain flexibility in the ankle and prevent permanent stiffness

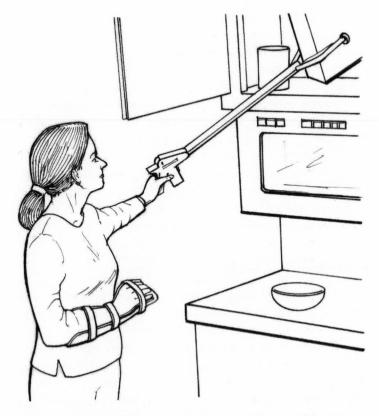

FIGURE 18.5   *Wrist/hand splint and reacher.*
A resting wrist/hand splint is used to position the weakened upper limb. A
reacher is used to grasp objects on the floor or, in this case, on a high shelf.

("contracture"). In cases of severe increases in muscle tone, a custom
splint can be fabricated by a physical therapist (generally a removable
two-piece fiberglass cast or a lightweight plastic splint), or by an orthotist
(typically a plastic splint with foam padding).

Dressing Aids

Many devices have been created to assist with dressing, though usually
only a limited number are useful for a given person. Some, like shoes
with Velcro closures, are widely available in conventional stores. Others

may be found through catalogues or web sites for assistive devices (see Appendix). Lace-up shoes can be converted to shoes with Velcro closures by a cobbler, and a variety of other clothing can be made to close with Velcro by a seamstress. Elastic shoelaces allow conversion of lace-up shoes into slip-on shoes. Long-handled shoehorns may make donning shoes or braces easier. Dressing sticks are multipurpose devices that are often helpful (see Figure 18.4); "sock pullers" can help a person put on socks or stockings. In addition, hooks to help with buttons and a variety of other devices are available to make dressing easier. Long-handled reachers may be useful for accessing clothing on shelves; they can be helpful in the kitchen as well (see Figure 18.5). The list of assistive devices is nearly endless; check with a physician or occupational therapist to see which devices might be best for you or your loved one.

Environmental Control Units

Environmental control units are electronic devices intended to allow a profoundly disabled individual to control electric appliances in his environment. These units are needed by only a very small percentage of stroke survivors, but they are often enormously important for this small group. Individuals with severe brain stem strokes are the most likely stroke survivors to benefit from these devices, which are more commonly used for people with severe quadriplegia after spinal cord injury. These devices can be attached to telephones, intercoms, televisions, fans, and other appliances. Some of the simpler devices are broadly available commercially (for example, at Radio Shack or similar stores), whereas other, more complex devices are only available from specialized vendors (and may be quite expensive). When considering this type of device, family members should ask the rehabilitation team for a referral to a regional center that specializes in helping people select assistive technology and training them in its use.

19

Nontraditional Treatments

Marybeth is a sixty-nine-year-old yoga instructor who develops atrial fibrillation and a resulting stroke. Her physician prescribes Coumadin (warfarin) for prevention of another stroke. Despite an extensive program of rehabilitation, she has persistent weakness of her arm and needs a cane to walk. She is interested in trying a natural herbal supplement her friend has recommended, as well as acupuncture treatment. She is hesitant to discuss these treatments with her physician, however, for fear that he will be uninterested, disapprove, or even ridicule them. Her sister, who is a nurse, strongly encourages her to discuss these options with her physician, and Marybeth reluctantly does so. Contrary to her expectations, her physician is supportive and open to her use of nontraditional treatments, as long as they are safe and do not interfere with her medical therapies. Marybeth's physician expresses support for a trial of acupuncture, but advises against the use of the herbal supplement out of concern that it may interfere with Coumadin metabolism. Marybeth undergoes acupuncture and feels that her energy level is improved. She decides not to use the herbal supplement because of her physician's concerns. Are nontraditional treatments safe after a stroke? Do they help? Which ones are best for stroke survivors?

Stroke recovery is often incomplete, despite extensive rehabilitation. While medical science continues to progress, there are many areas, such as stroke recovery, where it doesn't yet offer cures. As a result, people who have had a stroke and their families are often interested in exploring "nontraditional" treatments, sometimes also referred to as complementary or alternative medicine. Although most of these treatments are, by definition, not proven and not widely accepted by the medical profession at large, they may be a reasonable option for someone who wants to seek treatment alternatives. Often, consumers adopt the attitude, "it couldn't hurt, and maybe it will help," a reasonable approach when faced with a condition for which conventional medicine does not offer a cure. Some individuals also have personal or philosophical preferences for natural or other nontraditional treatments.

Because alternative treatments encompass a very broad range of options, from meditation to acupuncture to energy healing, it is important that each treatment be evaluated individually. Advertisements for amazing cures for almost every problem, including stroke, are easily found in the checkout aisle of any grocery store. Some of these treatments, such as acupuncture for pain management, are widely accepted and well studied. Others, such as crystal therapy, may be benign but ineffective. Still others, such as certain herbal treatments, may actually be dangerous in some cases. Here are some general rules of thumb when considering nontraditional treatments:

- Know the risks, reported benefits, and costs.
- Don't use nontraditional treatments as a replacement for important medical treatments (such as medications to prevent a second stroke).
- Make certain your physician is aware of all nontraditional treatments you are considering, and verify that they will not interfere or interact with conventional medical treatments.
- Avoid treatments with unrealistic or impossible claims ("cures stroke," and so on).

Acupuncture

Acupuncture is a long-established treatment that originated in China and has become popular as a treatment around the world. Although most acupuncture treatments share similar techniques such as insertion of fine needles and the use of electric stimulation through needles (electroacupuncture), there are actually many different approaches and nuances that have been developed in different regions. Many acupuncturists also offer related treatments, such as acupressure, moxabustion,

low-intensity laser acupuncture, and traditional Chinese herbal remedies. Most individuals in the United States receive acupuncture from
nonphysician acupuncturists, though some physicians are also trained
in this technique. Acupuncture has been best studied for pain treatment
and appears to be effective in certain types of pain conditions. It is less
well studied, though widely used, for promoting recovery after stroke.
The scientific studies of acupuncture post-stroke have had mixed results,
with some suggesting that it may be effective in stimulating recovery,
and others showing no significant effect. No studies have found evidence
of harm, and it appears that acupuncture is generally safe after stroke.
Acupuncture has also been anecdotally reported to temporarily reduce
spasticity after stroke, though this effect has not been carefully studied.
Since acupuncture has been found helpful for a variety of painful conditions, it may be particularly useful for stroke-related pain problems, such
as shoulder pain or central pain syndromes.

Individuals who take Coumadin (warfarin) should inform their physician and acupuncturist about this treatment, though acupuncture can
probably be used if the Coumadin dose is stable and the INR level appropriate. Individuals with pacemakers should avoid electroacupuncture,
which may interfere with pacemaker function.

Herbal Remedies

The contents of nutritional supplements and herbal remedies are not
standardized in the same way conventional medications are, adding to
the challenges faced by consumers. Potencies of botanical extracts are
not standardized and may vary substantially from one brand to another.
Because the marketing of these treatments is so varied, it is often difficult to ascertain exactly what treatment is being provided, and what
dose is contained in a capsule.

The reality is that some of these supplements are as powerful as prescription medications, and others are no more potent than a Lifesaver
candy. As with supplements, many conventional medications have their
origins in plant or other natural sources, including medications derived
from molds (penicillin), willow tree bark (aspirin), and yew shrubs (the
cancer treatment Taxol). These powerful treatments have been well re-

searched and tested, and complementary medications must be approached with the same respect and caution.

From the perspective of the stroke survivor, the major concern of these medications is their potential side effects, which may increase the risk of stroke or interfere with other, prescribed medications. Supplements containing ephedra may elevate blood pressure and should be avoided. Excessive vitamin K in a vitamin supplement can interfere with Coumadin's ability to protect against future stroke. No herbal treatments or nutritional supplements have been proven to help improve stroke recovery or prevent future strokes.

Stroke survivors should treat all supplements and herbal treatments as medicines, and not take any without consulting their physician. Given that many physicians are unfamiliar with these treatments and their brand names, it may be helpful to bring the actual container to a medical appointment before starting the supplement, so that the physician can evaluate its contents.

Vitamins

Vitamin supplements are on the boundary between nontraditional treatments and conventional medicine. Certain vitamins, such as folate, vitamin B6, and vitamin B12, have recently been proposed to reduce the risk of stroke by lowering homocysteine levels. While this still remains to be proven, some physicians are now advising their patients to take these vitamins while awaiting the results of studies to evaluate their efficacy. Other vitamins (for example, large doses of vitamin C) are sometimes used by individuals but do not have strong support in the scientific literature. Again, vitamin K interferes with the action of Coumadin (warfarin) and should not be used by stroke survivors unless advised by their physicians.

Hyperbaric Oxygen

Hyperbaric oxygen has been promoted as a treatment for aphasia or weakness after stroke but has not been rigorously tested. Most physicians consider this a speculative treatment for chronic stroke-related impairments. Hyperbaric oxygen is generally well tolerated, though it is not without risks and can be quite expensive. In general, hyperbaric oxygen therapy should be avoided after stroke until further research is conducted.

Osteopathic/Chiropractic Manipulation

Manipulation of the spine, performed by chiropractors and some osteopathic physicians, is used to treat a number of disorders, most prominently back and neck pain. Unfortunately, cervical spinal manipulation has been found to be a *cause* of a small number of strokes due to damage of the arteries in the neck (arterial dissection). Spinal manipulation should therefore be avoided by anyone with a history of arterial dissection. Since stroke survivors may suffer from back, neck, or other pain, manipulation is sometimes used to treat these unrelated conditions after stroke, and less commonly, to treat problems directly related to a stroke. There is no published research on its use after stroke, and no strong reason to believe that it is particularly helpful or harmful.

Therapeutic Massage

Massage therapy may be useful for certain types of muscle pain. Some individuals with spasticity (increased muscle tone) after stroke report reduced symptoms after massage, though this effect has not been studied scientifically. Deep-friction massage may cause bruising in people taking blood thinners like Coumadin and should be avoided. Other, more gentle forms of massage therapy should not generally pose any particular risk after stroke. As with any treatment, check with your doctor first.

Magnets

Magnets are sometimes used as a treatment for pain and other conditions. There is little scientific evidence to support their use generally, but little evidence of risk. Individuals with implanted medical devices such as pacemakers may experience interference from magnets and should avoid their use unless specifically discussed with their physician.

Homeopathy

Homeopathy is a form of alternative medicine whose central philosophy is that "like cures like," and that natural treatments should be designed to accentuate bodily responses to disease rather than "fight" them. Furthermore, homeopathy holds that the more a medication is diluted, the more powerful it becomes. Conventional medical practitioners (sometimes referred to as "allopathic physicians") are generally dubious that homeopathic treatments have any discernible effects, since they are extraordinarily dilute. While homeopathic treatments have not been proven effective in scientific studies, they are probably safe in most cases after stroke.

Biofeedback

Some forms of biofeedback, such as EMG (muscle) biofeedback for weakness after stroke, have been widely used as medical treatments and do not fall into the category of "alternative" treatments. These uses of EMG biofeedback are discussed in Chapter 11. Other forms of biofeedback, such as EEG (brainwave) biofeedback, remain highly controversial and are not widely accepted by conventional medical practitioners. These techniques appear safe but are of unproven efficacy after stroke.

Electrical Stimulation

Electrical stimulation of muscles to enhance movement, sometimes known as "functional electrical stimulation," or FES, is a technique that has been studied extensively in the medical and scientific community. Please see the discussion of this technique in Chapter 11.

Meditation

Meditation includes a variety of techniques for improved self-awareness and control of emotional states. These techniques are not well studied but are considered safe for individuals after stroke. They may be useful as an adjunctive treatment for spasticity, which is known to increase during times of anxiety or emotional upset.

Tai Chi

Tai chi is a long-established Chinese form of exercise primarily used to maintain health, but also used after illness or injury in some cases. This technique of slow, controlled movements and breathing emphasizes proper form. Tai chi has been found helpful for some individuals to prevent falls related to Parkinson's Disease, as well as for frail seniors to help them avoid falls. Although it has not been specifically studied after stroke, it may be a useful exercise technique for selected individuals. Given its slow and controlled movements, there are few safety concerns regarding the use of this technique.

Craniosacral Treatment

Craniosacral treatment is based on the belief that there are connections between the head and the lower spine (sacrum) that govern symptoms and energy flow through the body. Subtle movements between the bones of the skull or sacral bones are proposed to have far-ranging effects in the body. Craniosacral techniques are employed by some physical and occupational therapists as well as by other practitioners. While the efficacy of these techniques is debated and unproven, they involve gentle massage and movements and should be safe for someone who has had a stroke.

Yoga, Feldenkrais, and Other Exercise Techniques

There are many popular exercise techniques whose scientific effect poststroke have been studied very little, if at all. Most of these techniques are safe and reasonable options to try after stroke for the interested individual.

Aromatherapy

Aromatherapy involves the use of specific aromas that are claimed to be therapeutic, usually in promoting relaxation. Although there is no proof that this treatment is effective, there are no safety concerns regarding the use of aromatherapy after stroke.

Therapeutic Touch

Therapeutic touch is a controversial treatment involving the use of heal-ing energy fields transmitted from the healthcare practitioner to the pa-tient. These fields are not detectable using scientific techniques, and the presence of healing effects is unproven. Therapeutic touch is usually practiced without actual physical contact; rather, the practitioner places her hands close to the person she is treating. Although there is no scien-tific evidence that therapeutic touch is helpful after stroke, there is no reason to believe that it is in any way harmful. It may be used without concern for medical side effects.

There are many other forms of complementary and alternative medicine, and new approaches become available all the time. Stroke survivors are strongly advised to discuss these treatments with a physician before un-dertaking them, to prevent any interference or interactions with conven-tional medical treatments. Complementary and alternative medicine is best used as an adjunct to conventional medicine rather than as a substi-tute. Interested readers are directed to a text entitled *Complementary and Alternative Medicine in Rehabilitation* (see Appendix).

20

Understanding Clinical Research

Richard is a seventy-nine-year-old widower who is approached by a research assistant during his stay at a rehabilitation hospital after a stroke.
The research assistant explains that Richard may be eligible to participate
in a study of a new medication proposed to promote recovery after stroke.
Although he is interested in recovering as fully as possible, Richard is concerned about the possible risks of taking an untested medication, and he
doesn't want to be a "guinea pig." He has been given a nine-page, single-
spaced consent form to review, and he asks his daughter to help him understand the study and make a decision. How can she help Richard make
an informed decision regarding participation in this study?

Medical research is the engine that moves medical science forward.
Because of the natural variability in stroke severity and recovery, studies
of possible new treatments for stroke require testing in relatively large
groups of people to determine whether or not they are effective.

As medical research has grown, it has spread outside the traditional
large academic medical centers and can now be found in community
hospitals and private physician offices. Research in stroke is growing,
with a new emphasis on interventions to enhance recovery and rehabilitation. As a result, individuals who have had a stroke are more likely than
ever to be invited to participate in research studies. Although medical research is critical to advancing the treatment of stroke, the stroke survivor
and his family must carefully consider each individual study before making a decision to participate. The risks and benefits of research vary
widely, as do the personal perspectives and values of participants. Medical research is designed to answer scientific questions rather than benefit

the individual participants in the study. People are often motivated to participate in a clinical study out of the hope that it may help them personally. Although understandable, this desire for personal gain must be tempered with a realistic understanding of the nature of the study, as well as the risks and possible benefits to the individual participant. Alternatives to participation in the study should be fully understood as well.

Research can be categorized in several different ways. For the purposes of this book I have approached research studies from a potential subject's perspective. Under this rubric there are two broad categories of research: studies that involve treatment and those that do not.

Observational and Natural History Studies

Studies that do not test a specific medication or other medical treatment are most commonly natural history or observational studies. These studies are designed to gain a better understanding of the course of an illness, of the likelihood that a particular population will develop a medical condition, or of the outcome of a medical treatment that is being provided in the normal course of medical care. The information gathered through observational studies serves as an important first step in designing better treatments. Although these studies do not include new medical treatments, they may involve diagnostic testing of participants. This testing can vary from the trivial (such as an interview or physical examination) to extensive or invasive medical testing (for example, a cardiac catheterization). In observational studies, subjects may be examined or tested once or repeatedly. Examples of this type of research include a study using a new imaging technique of the brain to better understand the anatomical aspects of certain stroke symptoms, or a study that performs repeated language testing over the course of recovery from aphasia in order to understand the process by which aphasia improves over time.

Risk Factors

Similar in many ways to a natural history study, a study to determine risk factors is also an observational study, but with an emphasis on understanding who will develop an illness over time. Testing of participants for various characteristics that are suspected of being risk factors for a condition (for example, stroke) is an important part of these studies. These studies are usually low risk. Although they provide little potential benefit to the individual participant, they can be very helpful to future patients and may assist in the development of new treatments. Participation in this type of research is essentially an act of altruism, since there are no anticipated personal benefits.

Clinical Trials

Studies that assess the benefits of a medical treatment are often referred to as "clinical trials." These test the utility of a new or existing treatment in preventing or treating a medical condition. Clinical trials come in several varieties, often depending on how advanced the research is for a proposed treatment. The earliest studies of a proposed new treatment may assess the treatment effects and safety in an "open label" fashion; that is, with the participant and researchers fully aware of the exact nature of the subjects' treatment. These studies are generally not considered very informative about efficacy (whether a treatment works), but they can provide useful information about the appropriate dose of medication and how well people tolerate the treatment. From the subject's perspective, these studies may provide an early opportunity to receive a new treatment that may otherwise be unavailable. While this opportunity may allow participants to benefit from the treatment, it also puts them at risk of developing side effects or complications from a treatment that has not been studied very well yet. Furthermore, many treatments studied in this fashion prove useless, or worse—even harmful.

If preliminary studies show that a new treatment is reasonably safe and suggest that it may be effective, larger clinical trials may be conducted. Larger trials often compare a treatment to a "placebo" treatment; that is, to a "fake" treatment that is not believed to produce the desired clinical effect. These studies are often referred to as "placebo-controlled" studies. For medication studies, placebos are usually pills containing inert ingredients (such as a small amount of sugar) and are the same shape and color as the active treatment under study. In a device study, a placebo may look the same as the active device, though it does not actually deliver any treatment. In a placebo-controlled study, the research subjects are not told whether they are receiving the active treatment or the placebo. In many studies, the investigators themselves are not aware of which treatment each subject is receiving until the study is completed. If neither the participants nor the investigators know who is receiving which treatment, the study is known as a "double-blind placebo-controlled" study— the "gold standard" of clinical research.

Why do scientists use placebos and prevent participants from knowing which treatment they are receiving? Researchers have found that many conditions seem to improve when treated, regardless of whether the treatment actually has any biological effect. For example, a certain percentage (perhaps 30 percent) of people will feel better after receiving an inert pill for a headache. (Interestingly, placebos can also cause side effects, such as stomach upset and dizziness, among others.) Because of this placebo response, a new treatment may appear useful even if it is only causing a placebo effect. Although we still don't completely understand what causes a placebo effect, researchers have learned to account for this effect by intentionally giving some research participants an inert pill. They then compare the improvement in the placebo group to the improvement among subjects receiving an active treatment. If the active treatment provides a larger therapeutic benefit than the placebo treatment, then the treatment being tested is considered effective.

In most placebo-controlled studies, participants are randomly assigned to receive either the treatment being tested (the active treatment) or a placebo. Sometimes, a new treatment will be compared to an existing treatment rather than to a placebo treatment, or several different treatment regimens will be compared. Researchers should disclose to prospective participants the likelihood of their receiving each type of treatment so they can take this information into account when making a decision regarding participation.

In most clinical trials, the participants are not informed of their treatment assignment. The use of "blinding" (keeping participants and researchers from knowing treatment assignment) is important in a placebo-controlled study. Although this blinding may seem unfair to the research study participant, it is very important to the scientific design of the study and generally unavoidable. If study participants know that the placebo contains inert ingredients, their expectations of treatment failure might influence the results. Similarly, if the researchers are aware of which treatment each subject is receiving, this knowledge may unconsciously bias their interpretation of the effects of the treatments. Keeping both the participants and the researchers "in the dark" protects the study from unwitting bias. In some cases, treatment assignment cannot be hidden from the participant (for example, studies of certain exercise treatments) and thus blinding is not used.

Some researchers will disclose the nature of the treatment provided to individual participants after their participation has ended, or after the completion of the study. Others will provide participants with a synopsis of the results of the study at the conclusion, so that they can share in the knowledge that they helped create. Prospective participants should inquire about the availability of this information when deciding whether or not to enroll in a research study.

Sometimes clinical trials examine the potential benefits of a treatment that is already available but is not widely used or is of uncertain efficacy. In these situations, it may be possible for people to receive this treatment outside a research study. If the treatment is particularly appealing, a stroke survivor may prefer to seek this treatment outside a clinical trial to make certain that he is not assigned to a placebo.

Clinical Trials for Stroke

Clinical trials related to stroke treatment tend to fall into four major groups, depending on which aspect of stroke is being addressed. Stroke studies may address prevention, acute treatment, sub-acute treatment, or recovery and rehabilitation. These divisions are somewhat arbitrary, and treatments may overlap in two or more of these categories.

STROKE PREVENTION

Primary prevention. These are studies designed to prevent a first stroke from occurring. A primary prevention study might, for example, look at the use of aspirin or a cholesterol-lowering drug in a group of people at increased risk for stroke. These studies may involve new treatments for individuals known to benefit from existing treatments (such as an alternative to aspirin for stroke prevention), the use of an existing medication in individuals for whom the benefits of treatment are uncertain, or the potential benefits of exercise, diet modification, or other lifestyle modifications to prevent stroke.

Secondary prevention. These are studies of stroke prevention in people who have already had a stroke. Such a study might compare two medications that prevent blood-clot formation, or evaluate the effects of a medication to lower blood levels of a factor suspected to increase the risk of recurrent stroke (for example, homocysteine or cholesterol). When considering participating in such a study, stroke survivors should determine if an established treatment will be given to the control subjects or if a placebo treatment will be given instead.

ACUTE STROKE TREATMENT

Stroke damages the brain very quickly. Treatment with clot-dissolving medications such as intravenous alteplase (Activase) has been found to be most effective and safest if given within three hours after the onset of stroke symptoms. This is a very narrow window of opportunity, and many investigational treatments for acute stroke have a similarly narrow time frame. As such, there may be very limited time for a discussion of the pros and cons of an experimental treatment. Family members should make certain that they clearly understand the alternatives to participation in the study. Specifically, what treatment would be provided if participation in the study were declined? Is your family member a candidate for thrombolytic treatment (clot-busting medications such as alteplase)? Is this a placebo-controlled study? Unfortunately, there may not be time to research the proposed treatment or alternatives, making it all the more critical for the stroke patient and/or her family to have a discussion with the researcher to be sure they understand the risks and benefits of the proposed treatment. Among stroke studies, this type of study is most likely to carry both high risks and potentially large benefits.

SUB-ACUTE STROKE TREATMENT

The period of time beginning a few hours after a stroke and lasting for a few days after the stroke may be considered the sub-acute period. Researchers are seeking treatments that can be given during this time to reduce the neurological damage caused by stroke, or to stimulate recovery early after stroke. The time boundaries between acute stroke treatment, sub-acute treatment, and stroke recovery and rehabilitation are not clearly established, and some overlap exists.

STROKE RECOVERY AND REHABILITATION

Research on techniques to enhance stroke recovery has recently captured considerable attention among consumers and healthcare providers. Studies have shown that specialized exercises and activities appear to enhance motor abilities after stroke. Constraint Induced Movement Therapy (CIMT) is one prominent example of this type of research. Studies of stroke recovery and rehabilitation may also include medication studies, such as ongoing studies of dextroamphetamine, a medication proposed to enhance motor recovery after stroke. These studies are usually of low to moderate risk and are frequently conducted in a rehabilitation hospital unit or in the outpatient setting.

Locating a Clinical Trial

In some cases, a research team will directly contact you or your family member in the hospital or clinic to invite participation in a research study. In other cases, researchers will place advertisements in local newspapers or other locations to attract study participants. In many cases, however, participation in a clinical trial may require a search on the part of the individual or her family.

Many research studies are conducted at major academic hospitals (including rehabilitation hospitals), and contacting these institutions in your area will often identify studies of interest. Your family member's neurologist or physiatrist may be aware of studies in the region and should be contacted for information and possible referral. Internet registries of clinical research can be helpful (see Appendix), though these lists are often incomplete and may not be up-to-date. Research studies tend to be clustered in major metropolitan areas, and access to these opportunities may be limited outside these areas. Ultimately, a certain amount of detective work is often needed to find research of interest to your family member seeking innovative treatments after a stroke.

Deciding to Participate in a Clinical Trial

How should an individual make a decision regarding his own or a family member's participation in a clinical trial? Several factors should be considered. First, how good are the existing treatments for this condition? The reality is that current treatments for the after-effects of stroke, such as weakness, sensory loss, or aphasia, are still far from perfect. In the setting of an acute stroke, treatments are often limited or carry significant risk, as with thrombolysis (clot-dissolving treatment). In these circumstances, it is logical to consider participating in a study that may offer a new, alternative treatment that may be more effective than established treatments, safer, or both. This decision needs to be made on a case-by-case basis since not every proposed new treatment proves to be safe or effective, and there are benefits to using the established treatments, in spite of their limitations.

Second, what are the individual benefits to the study participant? Often they are minimal. An example would be a study of a new antihypertensive (blood pressure-reducing) medication for someone whose blood pressure can be safely controlled with other medications. Many of the existing treatments for hypertension are highly effective, well tolerated, and inexpensive. Here the only real benefits may be to future patients who may do well on this particular medication. One unfortunate phenomenon is the continued development of "me too" drugs by the pharmaceutical industry. In these cases, a safe and effective medication may exist, but competing drug companies want to develop their own version of the medication to sell in the marketplace. Sometimes these new medications have benefits beyond the existing medications, but all too often these "new" medications are essentially the same as the existing ones. Participating in studies of these medications may be more likely to help the pharmaceutical company than the individual participant or future patients.

Third, who is sponsoring a study? Often this information can provide additional insights into the nature of the research. Most clinical research in the United States is sponsored by the pharmaceutical industry, the government (primarily through the National Institutes of Health, or NIH), and charitable foundations. NIH-sponsored studies are subjected to a very rigorous review process and tend to be well designed from a scientific perspective. Pharmaceutical-sponsored research (or research sponsored by another commercial enterprise, such as a device manufacturer) is usually designed to answer questions of commercial interest to the sponsoring company. These studies tend to be carefully designed, though prospective participants should scrutinize the proposed benefits to avoid participating in a "me too" study of a new treatment that really just duplicates an existing treatment. Research sponsored by charitable foundations is quite diverse and may include some newer treatment approaches that have not yet been extensively studied. Ultimately, it is the specific aspects of the research rather than the sponsorship that should inform a decision whether or not to participate in a research study.

WHAT TO ASK?

When considering a particular research study, potential participants (or their families) should ask the following key questions:

- What are the risks of this study? Has this medication or treatment been tried in other human studies? What was found?
- What types of side effects are likely? What serious side effects or complications might occur? What is the likelihood that these complications will occur?
- Can I decide to participate in this study at a later date?
- What benefits are the researchers hoping to find? Do they expect large improvements in function, or small differences? Will this effect be enough to impact my ability to perform daily tasks?
- What alternative treatments are available? What treatment will be provided if I don't participate in the study? Is the study treatment available outside of a research study?
- Is there a placebo group? What are my chances of receiving the active treatment? If I am assigned to the placebo group, can I receive the experimental treatment after completion of the study?
- Has this study been approved by an Institutional Review Board (IRB)? How can I contact the IRB if I have any questions or concerns with the conduct of the study?
- How will my confidentiality be maintained?
- Who will be available for any questions or problems that develop? How do I contact that person?

- What happens if I have any side effects or complications?
- What treatment is available in the event of a complication? Who will pay for it?
- Are there any costs associated with participating? Will my insurance company be billed for any costs?
- How can I find out the results of this study if I choose to participate?

Some studies compensate participants for their time and inconvenience. In other studies, reimbursement for parking and transportation expenses may be available if requested. Remember that research participants are helping the researcher as much as the researcher is helping the participants.

Research Subject Rights

As a participant in a research study, you or your family member has certain rights. These include the right to receive a thorough explanation of risks, benefits, and alternatives to participating in the study, to withdraw from the study at any time, to be notified of any new treatments or information that become available during the course of participation in the study that might impact a decision to continue participation, and others. Each institution conducting clinical research is required either to have a special research committee known as the Institutional Review Board, or to contract with another institution to provide this review. The role of this board is to review all research studies involving human subjects and ensure that subjects' rights are appropriately protected. Research participants should be provided with contact information for the IRB should any questions or complaints arise regarding their rights as research participants.

Many larger studies that pose significant risks to subjects also have a safety review board that monitors any adverse events that occur in study participants. Interim analyses of study results are often done during the study to ensure that no group of subjects is experiencing adverse outcomes as a result of the study.

Recent federal regulations under the Health Information Portability and Accountability Act (HIPAA) provide new protections for the privacy of health information, and research studies have specific requirements under this new set of regulations. Further information regarding the protections provided under this act are available at government web sites (see Appendix).

Given the complexity of the information and decision-making process, family involvement is often critical in decisions regarding participation in a research study. Unless the study has a very narrow window for enrollment (for example, an acute-stroke treatment), insist on taking sufficient time to review the information provided. Make certain you ask questions. This is the best guarantee of a favorable experience when participating in clinical research.

Resources and Information

This list contains information on a variety of public and private resources. Inclusion in this list does not imply endorsement of any service or product.

General Information about Stroke (see also Stroke Organizations below)

Cerebral Amyloid Angiopathy Web Site
A web site devoted to cerebral amyloid angiopathy research and education.
www.angiopathy.org

Massachusetts General Hospital Department of Neurology
Web page provides information about stroke prevention and treatment, and hosts an on-line support/discussion group on stroke.
dem0nmac.mgh.harvard.edu

Massachusetts General Hospital Department of Neurosurgery
Web page provides extensive information on treatment of vascular abnormalities (aneurysms, arteriovenous malformations, carotid stenosis) causing stroke.
neurosurgery.mgh.harvard.edu/neurovascular

MedlinePlus Health Information
A free service sponsored by the National Library of Medicine and the National Institutes of Health, providing information about health con-

ditions and medications, a health encyclopedia and glossary with pictures and diagrams, and health news.
www.nlm.nih.gov/medlineplus

Stroke: Your Complete Exercise Guide
by Neil F. Gordon
A guide to exercise after stroke.
Human Kinetics, 1993
ISBN: 0-873-22428-0

Washington University in St. Louis Internet Stroke Center
Web resource provides information about stroke, with links to directory of stroke research studies and other resources.
www.strokecenter.org

Community Resources

Elder Services
The eldercare locator is run by the U.S. Administration on Aging and provides links to a wide variety of state and local resources for older individuals.
1-800-677-1116
www.eldercare.gov

Complementary and Alternative Medicine

Complementary and Alternative Medicine in Rehabilitation
Edited by Eric Leskowitz, M.D., and Marc S. Micozzi, M.D.
A medical textbook on the use of alternative medicine in rehabilitation.
Churchill Livingstone, 2002
ISBN: 0-443-06599-3

Devices and Services

Abledata
A federally funded project to provide information on assistive technology and rehabilitation equipment available from domestic and interna-

tional sources to consumers, organizations, professionals, and caregivers within the United States.
8630 Fenton Street
Suite 930 Silver Spring, MD 20910
(301) 608-8998; or 1-800-227-0216 (8:00 A.M.–5:30 P.M. ET)
TTY: (301) 608-8912
fax: (301) 608-8958
www.abledata.com

Guldmann, Inc.
Manufacturer of ceiling lifts to assist with mobility for the disabled, as
well as other mobility systems.
5505 Johns Road
Suite 700
Tampa, FL 33634
(813) 880-0619; or 1-800-664-8834
fax: (813) 880-9558
e-mail: info@guldmann.net
www.guldmann.com

Hocoma AG
Manufacturer of the Lokomat robot, which provides walking exercises
after stroke and other conditions.
Florastrasse 47
CH-8008, Zurich
Switzerland
phone: 41-1-380-57-37
fax: 41-1-380-57-38
e-mail: info@hocoma.ch
www.hocoma.ch/engl/index.html

Independence Technology (Johnson & Johnson)
Manufacturer and distributor of the iGLIDE wheelchair (manual wheelchair with power assist) and the iBOT power wheelchair with advanced
mobility features (able to climb stairs, and so on).
(877) 794-4588
www.iglidenow.com

Interactive Motion Technologies (IMT)
Manufacturer of the InMotion 2 robot, which provides arm exercises
after stroke. Research is ongoing with this robot at a number of centers
in the United States.
56 Highland Avenue
Cambridge, MA 02139
(617) 497-6330
fax: 617-864-3829
e-mail: info@interactive-motion.com
interactive-motion.com

Novavision
Provider of a computer-based retraining system for visual field loss resulting from stroke and other causes. This system will soon be available
in the United States.
Hansapark 1
39120 Magdeburg Germany
tel.: 0391-63-600-50
fax: 0391-63-600-70
www.nanopharm.de/novaeng.html

Stroke Recovery Systems, Inc.
Distributor of the Neuromove system, which provides combined biofeedback and functional electrical stimulation for post-stroke weakness.
4 West Dry Creek
Circle Suite 260
Denver, CO 80120
www.strokeaid.com

ZYGO Industries, Inc.
Manufacturer of assistive devices for communication disorders, including the Lightwriter keyboard/speech synthesis device.
P.O. Box 1008
Portland, OR 97207-1008
(503) 684-6006; or 1-800-234-6006
fax: (503) 684-6011
e-mail: zygo@zygo-usa.com
www.zygo-usa.com

Diet and Dysphagia

The American Heart Association Cookbook, 25th Anniversary Edition
A heart- and stroke-healthy cookbook. The American Heart Association also produces low-salt, low-calorie, and low-fat/low-cholesterol cookbooks.
Random House, Inc.
ISBN: 0-609-80890-7

Non-Chew Cookbook
by Wilson J. Randy
A cookbook for individuals with chewing and swallowing disorders. Sample recipes are posted on the book's web site.
Wilson Publishing, Inc.
P.O. Box 912464
Sherman, TX 75091
1-800-843-2409
www.nonchewcookbook.com

Vitamin K Web Site
The Dupont web site (makers of Coumadin brand warfarin) provides an extensive listing of the vitamin K content of various foods for warfarin users.
www.coumadin.com/consumer/INT_VitaminK1.asp

Disability Resources

Disability Exchange
A web service providing information for individuals with disabilities.
www.disabilityexchange.org

Disability Info
A federally sponsored web site providing links to a broad range of resources for people with disabilities.
disabilityinfo.gov

Easter Seals
A charitable organization that provides services to children and adults with disabilities and other special needs, and support to their families.

Many state chapters provide help with assistive technology and stroke support groups.
230 West Monroe Street, Suite 1800
voice: (312) 726-6200; or 1-800-221-6827
TTY: (312) 726-4258
fax: (312) 726-1494
www.easter-seals.org

National Council on Disability

A government agency advising the President and Congress on issues affecting people with disabilities.
1331 F Street, NW
Suite 850
Washington, DC 20004
(202) 272-2004
TTY: (202) 272-2074
fax: (202) 272-2022

National Rehabilitation Information Center (NARIC)

A federally supported resource center for information regarding disability and rehabilitation.
4200 Forbes Boulevard
Suite 202
Lanham, MD 20706
voice: (301) 459-5900; or 1-800-346-2742
e-mail: naricinfo@heitechservices.com
www.naric.com

Driving

Association for Driver Rehabilitation Specialists (ADED)

A professional organization of driver rehabilitation instructors. Web site provides a nationwide directory of driver rehabilitation specialists.
711 S. Vienna Street
Ruston, LA 71270
(318) 257-5055; or 1-800-290-2344
fax: (318) 255-4175
www.driver-ed.org

Emergency Response Systems

Commercial services that provide emergency alert systems for individuals who are at home alone and who have difficulty communicating, or are at risk for falls.

LifeFone, Inc.
1-800-882-2280
www.lifefone.com

LifeLine, Inc.
111 Lawrence Street
Framingham, MA 01702-8156
1-800-451-0525
fax: (508) 988-1384
e-mail: info@lifelinesys.com
www.lifelinesys.com

Organizations for Caregivers

Family Caregiver Alliance
An organization promoting the development of policies and programs for caregivers.
690 Market Street
Suite 600
San Fancisco, CA 94104
(415) 434-3388; or 1-800-445-8106
fax: (415) 434-3508
e-mail: info@caregiver.org
www.caregiver.org

National Family Caregivers Association
A family caregiver advocacy, support, and education organization.
10400 Connecticut Ave. no. 500
Kensington, MD 20895-3944
(800) 896-3650
fax: 301-942-2302
e-mail: info@nfcacares.org
www.nfcacares.org

Rosalyn Carter Institute for Human Development
An institute promoting research, education, and training in caregiver issues; also involved in advocacy efforts.
800 Wheatley Street
Americus, GA 31709
(229) 928-1234
fax: (229) 931-2663
e-mail: rci@rci.gsw.edu
www.rci.gsw.edu

Wellspouse Foundation
An association of spousal caregivers.
63 West Main Street
Suite H
Freehold, NJ 07728
1-800-838-0879
fax: (732) 577-8644
e-mail: info@wellspouse.org
www.wellspouse.org

Personal Accounts of Stroke and Recovery

After Stroke
by David M. Hinds and Peter Morris
Thorsons Publishing, 2000
ISBN: 0-722-53885-5

The Diving Bell and the Butterfly: A Memoir of Life in Death
by Jean-Dominique Bauby, trans. Jeremy Leggatt
A first-person account of living with "locked-in" syndrome.
Vintage Books, 1998
ISBN: 0-375-70121-4

My Stroke of Luck
by Kirk Douglas
A memoir by the well-known actor of his stroke and its aftermath.

William Morrow, 2002
ISBN: 0-060-00929-2

My Year Off: Recovering Life after a Stroke
by Robert McCrum
Broadway Books, 1999
ISBN: 0-767-90400-1

One-Handed in a Two-Handed World, 2nd ed.
by Tommye-Karen Mayer
A personal perspective on living with only one functional hand.
Prince-Gallison Press, Boston, 2000
ISBN: 0-965-28051-9

A Stroke of Genius: Messages of Hope and Healing from a Thriving Stroke Survivor
by Sandy Simon
Cedars Group, 2001
ISBN 0-966-96252-4

Your Mother Has Suffered a Slight Stroke
by Kathleen Bosworth
A caregiver's account of her mother's stroke and its impact.
Publish America, 2001
ISBN: 1-588-51288-6

Privacy Rights (HIPAA)

Health Insurance Portability and Accountability Act (HIPAA)
The U.S. Department of Health and Human Services—Office of Civil Rights provides information on its web site about the legal protections provided by this legislation.
www.hhs.gov/ocr/hipaa

Center for Medicare and Medicaid Services: HIPAA Information
United States Center for Medicare and Medicaid Services (CMS) official web site for HIPAA information.
cms.hhs.gov/hipaa/online/default.asp

Professional Organizations

American Academy of Physical Medicine and Rehabilitation

An organization for physicians specializing in physical medicine and re-habilitation. Information regarding this specialty, as well as an on-line directory of physiatrists, is available on the web site.

One IBM Plaza, Suite 2500
Chicago, IL 60611–3604
(312) 464-9700
e-mail: info@aapmr.org
fax: (312) 464-0227
www.aapmr.org

American Neurological Association

An organization of physicians specializing in neurology.
5841 Cedar Lake Road, Suite 204
Minneapolis, MN 55416
voice: (952) 545-6284
fax: (952) 545-6073
www.aneuroa.org

American Occupational Therapy Association

A national organization of occupational therapists.
4720 Montgomery Lane
P.O. Box 31220
Bethesda, MD 20824–1220
(301) 652-2682; or 1-800-377-8555
fax: (301) 652-7711
www.aota.org

American Physical Therapy Association

A national organization of physical therapists.
1111 North Fairfax Street
Alexandria, VA 22314
(703) 684-APTA (2782); or 1-800-999-APTA (2782)
TDD: (703) 683-6748
fax: (703) 684-7343
www.apta.org

American Society of Neurorehabilitation
An organization of neurologists and other physicians devoted to the rehabilitation of stroke and other neurological disorders.
5841 Cedar Lake Road, Suite 204
Minneapolis, MN 55416
(952) 545-6324
fax: (952) 545-6073
www.asnr.com

American Speech Language and Hearing Association
A national organization of speech language pathologists and audiolo-
gists.
10801 Rockville Pike
Rockville, MD 20852
voice/TTY: 1-800-638-8255 (8:30 A.M.–5:00 P.M. ET)
e-mail: actioncenter@asha.org.
www.asha.org

American Therapeutic Recreation Association
A national organization for recreation therapists.
1414 Prince Street, Suite 204
Alexandria, Virginia 22314
(703) 683-9420
fax: (703) 683-9431
www.atra-tr.org

Association of Rehabilitation Nurses
A national organization of nurses specializing in rehabilitation.
4700 W. Lake Avenue
Glenview, IL 60025-1485
(847) 375-4710; or 1-800-229-7530
fax: (877) 734-9384
e-mail: info@rehabnurse.org
www.rehabnurse.org

National Association of Professional Geriatric Care Managers
A national organization of community-based geriatric case managers.
1604 N. Country Club Road

Tucson, AZ 85716-3102
(520) 881-8008
fax: (520) 325-7925
www.caremanager.org

Rehabilitation Engineering and Assistive Technology Society of North America (RESNA)
An interdisciplinary association of professionals involved in helping people with disabilities through the use of technology.
1700 N. Moore St, Suite 1540
Arlington, VA 22209-1903
(703) 524-6686
TTY: (703) 524-6639
fax: (703) 524-6630
www.resna.org

Rehabilitation and Adaptive Equipment

Hutchinson Medical
333 Highland Avenue
Salem, MA
1-800-287-1770
www.hutchinsonmedical.com

Sammons Preston Rolyan
Provides an extensive on-line and conventional catalogue of aids to assist with mobility and activities of daily living.
4 Sammons Court
Bolingbrook, IL 60440
1-800-323-5547
fax: 1-800-547-4333
e-mail: sp@sammonspreston.com
www.sammonspreston.com

Rehabilitation Facilities

Commission for the Accreditation of Rehabilitation Facilities (CARF)
A nonprofit organization that provides accreditation to rehabilitation facilities on a voluntary basis.

4891 E. Grant Road
Tucson, AZ 85712
voice/TTY: (520) 325-1044
fax: (520) 318-1129
www.carf.org

HOME CARE AGENCIES

The Center for Medicare and Medicaid Services (CMS), a federal agency, provides on-line information on the outcomes achieved at home health agencies.
www.medicare.gov/HHCompare/Home.asp

SKILLED NURSING FACILITIES

The Center for Medicare and Medicaid Services (CMS), a federal agency, provides information on skilled nursing facility performance on a variety of measures on its web site.
www.medicare.gov/nhcompare/home.asp

Resources for Medical Professionals

The following resources are intended primarily for medical professionals but may be of interest to family members seeking to learn more about stroke and its consequences.

Journal of Stroke and Cerebrovascular Disease

A medical journal devoted to stroke and its treatment, published by the National Stroke Association.
www.strokejournal.org

National Institute of Neurological Disorders and Stroke (NINDS)

The U.S. government-sponsored center within the National Institutes of Health devoted to supporting research in stroke and other neurological disorders.
www.ninds.nih.gov

Pub Med

A free service provided by the National Library of Medicine that provides user-friendly searches of the medical literature for articles of inter-

est. Includes some summaries of articles (abstracts), as well as links to full texts of a limited array of articles.
www.ncbi.nlm.nih.gov/pubmed

Stroke
A medical journal devoted to prevention and treatment of stroke, published by the American Stroke Association (American Heart Association). Article titles and abstracts may be searched and reviewed without charge.
www.stroke.ahajournals.org

Return to Work

Mobility International USA (MIUSA)
A U.S.-based nonprofit organization devoted to empowering people with disabilities around the world through international exchange, information, technical assistance, and training. Works to ensure the inclusion of people with disabilities in international exchange and development programs.
P.O. Box 10767
Eugene, Oregon 97440
tel/TTY: (541) 343-1284
fax: (541) 343-6812
e-mail: info@miusa.org
www.miusa.org

Office of Special Education and Rehabilitative Services (OSERS)
The U.S. Department of Education, through OSERS, provides information and resources for vocational training and return to work for the disabled.
400 Maryland Avenue, SW
Washington, DC 20202
(202) 205-5465
www.ed.gov/offices/OSERS

State Vocational Rehabilitation Programs
Web site that provides a list of contact information for state vocational rehabilitation programs.
www.jan.wvu.edu/sbses/vocrehab.htm

U.S. Department of Justice Americans with Disabilities Act (ADA)
Web site provides an explanation of the ADA, answers to frequently
asked questions, and links to other resources regarding the rights of
peoples with disabilities.
1-800-514-0301
TDD: 1-800-514-0383
usdoj.gov/crt/ada/adahom1.htm

Sports and Leisure Activities

AccessSport America
A charitable organization that provides assistance with windsurfing,
kayaking, and other water sports for the disabled. Sponsors activities in
Massachusetts, New Hampshire, and Florida.
119 High Street
Acton, MA 01720
(866) 45-SPORT (77678); or (978) 264-0985
www.accessportamerica.org

Disabled Sports USA
A national organization whose chapters in more than thirty states support a broad range of sports activities, ranging from cycling and skiing
to sailing.
451 Hungerford Drive
Suite 100
Rockville, MD 20850
(301) 217-0960
fax: (301) 217-0968
www.dsusa.org

North American Riding for the Handicapped Association (NARHA)
A national organization that promotes horseback riding for individuals
with disabilities. Provides links to regional organizations.
P.O. Box 33150
Denver, CO 80233
(303) 452-1212; or 1-800-369-RIDE (7433)
fax: 303-252-4610

fax on demand: (303) 457-8496
e-mail: narha@narha.org
www.narha.org

Outdoor Explorations
An organization that provides organized outdoor activities for people
with disabilities and their families in the New England region.
98 Winchester Street
Medford, MA 02155
(781) 395-4999
TTY: (781) 395-4184
fax: (781) 395-4183
e-mail: info@outdoorexp.org
outdoorexp.org

United States Adaptive Golf Association
A national organization that promotes golf for individuals with
disabilities.
e-mail: golfpro@usagas.org
www.usagas.org

Stroke in Children

Blood Clots and Strokes: A Guide for Parents and Little Folks
by Maureen Andrew, M.D. A question-and-answer guide to childhood
stroke intended for parents.
BC Decker, 1998
ISBN: 1-550-09064-X

Children's Hemiplegia and Stroke Association (CHASA)
A nonprofit support organization for families of children with stroke.
Suite 305, PMB 149
4101 W. Green Oaks
Arlington, TX 76016
(817) 492-4325
e-mail: info5@chasa.org
www.chasa.org

The Pediatric Stroke Support Network
A family support organization providing information about stroke in children.
c/o Heather Tangen
P.O. Box 253
Greendale, WI 53129
e-mail: Heather@pediatricstrokenetwork.com
www.pediatricstrokenetwork.com

Stroke Clinical Research Resources

Centerwatch
A nationwide listing of clinical trials, organized geographically.
www.centerwatch.com

Clinical Research Network
Clinical research at a number of Harvard-affiliated hospitals in the Boston area.
crnet.mgh.harvard.edu/home/home.asp

NIH Clinical Trials Database
A searchable database containing information about clinical trials throughout the country, including those sponsored by the government, industry, and other sources.
clinicaltrials.gov

RehabTrials.org
A web site sponsored by the Kessler Medical Rehabilitation Research and Education Corporation, providing a listing of rehabilitation research studies.
www.rehabtrials.org

Stroke Trials Directory
A cooperative venture of the Internet Stroke Center at Washington University in St. Louis, the American Stroke Association, and the National Institute of Neurological Disorders and Stroke (National Institutes of Health), listing stroke research studies nationwide.
www.strokecenter.org/trials

Stroke Organizations (includes consumer and advocacy organizations)

American Stroke Association (A division of the American Heart Association)
A national organization devoted to the prevention and treatment of stroke.
National Center
7272 Greenville Avenue
Dallas, TX 75231
1-888-4-STROKE or 1-888-478-7653
www.strokeassociation.org

Brain Injury Association of America
A national advocacy organization for survivors of traumatic brain injury and their families. Provides information as well as links to state chapters of the organization and other resources.
105 North Alfred Street
Alexandria, VA 22314
family helpline: 1-800-444-6443
e-mail: familyhelpline@biausa.org.
www.biausa.org

Heart and Stroke Association of Canada
A organization devoted to improving the health of Canadians by preventing and reducing disability and death from heart disease and stroke through research, health promotion, and advocacy.
www.heartandstroke.ca

National Aphasia Association
An organization devoted to individuals with aphasia and their families.
1-800-922-4622
e-mail: naa@aphasia.org.
www.aphasia.org

National Stroke Association
A national organization devoted to the prevention and treatment of stroke.
9707 E. Easter Lane

Englewood, CO 80112
1-800-STROKES
303-649-9299
fax: 303-649-1328
www.stroke.org

The Stroke Association (United Kingdom)
A British national charity providing support for people who have had strokes, their families, and carers.
Stroke House
240 City Road
London, United Kingdom
EC1V 2PR
Telephone the Stroke Information Service on 020 7566 0330, or local rate number (from U.K.) 0845 30 33 100.
e-mail: info@stroke.org.uk
www.stroke.org.uk

Travel

Access-Able Travel Source
A web site devoted to helping individuals with disabilities locate travel resources. Includes links to travel agencies with expertise in meeting the needs of disabled travelers.
www.access-able.com

Accessible Journeys
A commercial travel agency specializing in providing customized trips for individuals with disabilities.
(610) 521-0339; or 1-800-846-4537
fax: (610) 521-6959
e-mail: sales@disabilitytravel.com
www.disabilitytravel.com/index.html

Disabled Travel Agency Directory
A web directory of travel agencies providing services for individuals with disabilities.
dmoz.org/Society/Disabled/Travel/Agencies

Flying Wheels, Inc.
A commercial travel agency specializing in meeting the travel needs of people with physical disabilities.
143 W. Bridge St.
P.O. Box 382
Owatonna, MN 55060
(507) 451-5005
fax: (507) 451-1685
www.flyingwheelstravel.com

Fodors
Web site includes tips for travelers with disabilities, as well as links to other travel resources.
www.fodors.com/traveltips/disabilities

Index